Providing Information
for Health

A workbook for primary care

Radcliffe Medical Press Ltd
18 Marcham Road
Abingdon
Oxon OX14 1AA
United Kingdom

www.radcliffe-oxford.com
The Radcliffe Medical Press electronic catalogue and on-line ordering facility.
Direct sales to anywhere in the world.

British Library Cataloguing in Publication Data

A catalogue record for this book is available from the British Library.

ISBN 1 85775 916 8

Typeset by Joshua Associates Ltd, Oxford
Printed and bound by TJ International Ltd, Padstow, Cornwall

Contents

About this book

A few years ago I wrote a book entitled *Information and IT for Primary Care* (Gillies, 1999a). My elder daughter refers to it as my cartoon book. I have been trying to write a book to follow on from my 'cartoon book' ever since.

This is that book. It is designed as a workbook. It covers 18 topics at the heart of *Information for Health*. Each topic gets its own chapter. They appear to vary in length, but this reflects the on-line resources called in to each topic. One of the shortest chapters in the book deals with the Bristol scandal; however, it does include on-line the 520-page Bristol inquiry report!

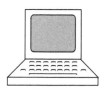

On-line resource

This book is actually half of a package. The other half is the Internet site. You will not enjoy reading this book unless you can access the accompanying website:

http://www.providinginformationforhealth.co.uk

In 1999, when I wrote *Information and IT for Primary Care* Internet access within the NHS was much less common than it is today. The Internet site for that book was an optional extra. For this book, it is an integral part of the whole.

Each time the book calls on an on-line resource you will see the computer symbol.

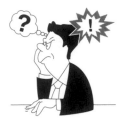 **Questions to think about**

All chapters include questions to think about. These provide a chance for reflection and reinforce key learning points in each chapter.

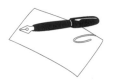 **Practical activities**

Many chapters have practical activities associated with them. These are designed to encourage you to take what you have learned from the book and apply it in your workplace.

 Key points

At the end of each chapter there are two or three key learning points to reinforce the most important issues for the reader to take away from that chapter.

And in keeping with the 'cartoon' tradition, many chapters start with one!

Alan Gillies
February 2002
professor@alangillies.co.uk

For Rachael and Anna.

1

Historical evolution

Introduction

This chapter will attempt to show how the current situation in primary and community healthcare informatics has arisen as a consequence of policy decisions made in the past.

History

Up until the late 1980s, GP computing was a minority sport. (Primary care informatics was unheard of.) The reforms implemented in the late 1980s and early 1990s, which resulted in fundholding, the new GP contracts and the internal markets, led amongst other things to a rapid growth in the number of computers found in general practice.

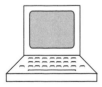

On-line resource
Now view the on-line poster, A comparison of the computerisation of medical practice in the public health sector, accessible in the Chapter 1 section of the website. This was presented in the USA in 1993 (Gillies, 1993).

I wrote the following account of the situation in 1995.

Introduction

This paper will consider the computerisation of primary healthcare in five sections:

- the area under scrutiny
- the methods and sources used
- the observations
- the issues identified
- conclusions.

The area under scrutiny

The UK family health sector

General medical practice is the part of the UK National Health Service (NHS) which patients encounter most often. Over the last seven years, there have been major changes in the organisation and working practices within this sector.

These changes were driven by a number of key pieces of Government legislation (Department of Health, 1986, 1987, 1989):

1986: Primary Care: an agenda for discussion
1987: Promoting Better Health, Government White Paper on Primary Care
1989: General Practice in the NHS: the 1990 Contract.

Prior to 1986, the role of the family doctor was seen as a provider of medicines to tackle simple diseases and a mechanism for referring more seriously ill patients to hospital.

The problem with this approach was the cost. Further, there were few checks on value for money and on the effectiveness of resource management. The NHS budget as a percentage of GDP has risen continually since the 1950s (*see* Figure 1.1).

In order to attempt to arrest this trend, Government policy laid down in the *Promoting Better Health* White Paper (Department of Health, 1987) set out the following aims:

- to focus upon preventive healthcare
- to require doctors to provide better information to the Family Health Service Authority (FHSA) in order to increase accountability
- to link doctors' incomes to performance measured against specific targets.

The reforms set out in these pieces of legislation divided the NHS into 'suppliers' and 'purchasers' with primary healthcare on the purchasing side and secondary healthcare on the supply side. This is known as the internal market within the NHS.

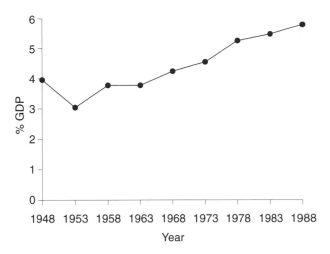

Figure 1.1 NHS budget as a percentage of GDP.
Source: Office of Health Economics, 1989.

Implementing this policy required doctors to improve their information systems dramatically, at the same time as absorbing change in just about every area of their working lives.

The administrative structure was also changed with the old style Family Practitioner Committees being replaced in England and Wales by FHSAs. These new bodies were given the ambiguous role of assisting doctors in the provision of primary healthcare whilst at the same time acting as quality monitors policing the new performance targets on behalf of the Government. In Scotland, the regional health boards (RHBs) remained responsible for the provision of family health alongside the hospital sector (*see* Figure 1.2).

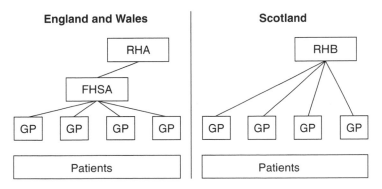

Figure 1.2 The role of FHSAs in England and Wales.

The situation was further complicated by the legislation which allows for the establishment of general practices with independent budgets for the purchase of external services, i.e. hospital beds for their patients. These doctors are known as 'fundholders'. On the supply side of the NHS marketplace, by 1994, most hospitals and other service providers in England and Wales had become trusts. These trusts are independent of the health authority and can supply services to almost anyone with a budget.

Under the new contractual arrangements, it is possible for doctors to assume control of their own budgets rather than remain under the budgetary control of the local FHSA.

One of the problems in trying to carry out this study is the diversity found in general practice. There is no typical model of delivering primary healthcare.

Within a medium size town of 100 000 inhabitants, one would expect to find about 60 family doctors with an average number of patients of 1670 per doctor. In such a town, one would expect to find a few large health centres where a complete service is offered including other health professionals such as practice nurses, therapists, opthalmists and even dentists. These would function alongside doctors working alone or in small units of two or three. Whereas during the 1960s and 1970s the trend was towards larger group practices, now there appears to be no discernible overall trend.

Certain factors, for example culture, do encourage particular modes of delivery. Single-practice doctors are prevalent in areas with a high proportion of the population from ethnic minorities.

The motivation for computerisation

The computerisation of general practice has been driven by the demands of Government legislation, specifically the 1987 White Paper, mentioned above and the introduction of new contracts and working conditions for GPs in 1990.

The emphasis on preventive care made specific demands for GPs to be able to identify groups of patients by age and sex as well as by clinical conditions. The obligation to provide an annual report further required the collection of data on referrals and on the use of external services.

A combination of 'carrot and stick' has led to a considerable increase in the uptake of technology. The doctors' incomes were tied to performance targets such as the percentage of children immunised, or the percentage of women screened for cervical cancer. The need to carry out these tasks and monitor performance dramatically increased the doctors' information requirements. This made the adoption of computers essential in the medium term and highly desirable in the immediate term. This formed the stick. The carrot offered was a 50% reimbursement of running expenses under the new contract.

The best national statistics available (Department of Health, Statistics and Management Information Division, 1989, 1990, 1993) show that this approach was highly effective in increasing the use of technology. In 1989, prior to the new contracts, 25% of doctors had installed computer-based information systems. Just one year later, in 1990, after the new contracts were introduced, this figure had doubled to 50%. The comparable figure in 1993 had risen to 79%.

Other surveys indicate a similar trend, but show discrepancies between studies due to regional variations.

Even within health regions there are great differences. For example in the North West of England, in the Lancashire FHSA area, the uptake of computers on the Fylde Coast, where healthcare is provided generally from group practices working from large health centres, is almost universal. In Blackburn where the stereotypical practice is single-handed and working in poor neighbourhoods with a large population from ethnic minorities, computer uptake is low and reliable data are difficult to establish.

In spite of some discrepancies in the figures there are two discernible features. The trend is inexorably upwards and there was an acceleration when the new contracts were announced in 1989 (*see* Figure 1.3).

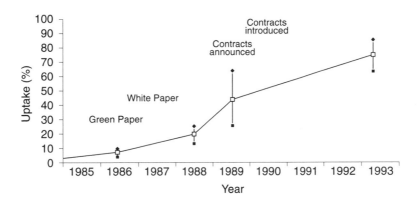

Figure 1.3 The installation of computer systems within general practice.

As an example, Salford FHSA, serving a generally poor catchment area which often corresponds to a slower uptake of computers, set 1994 as the target for 100% computerisation whereas other FHSAs had already reached this state.

Hayes (1985) identified the following barriers to the adoption of computers before the new contracts:

- incomplete coverage of all activities
- fears about confidentiality
- high average age of GPs (>60% over 40).

These may be compared to barriers found by a survey of GPs using computers after the imposition of new contracts (Shum, 1992):

- 66% of respondents found selecting systems to be a problem
- 49% had experienced difficulty using their systems
- 70% wanted to learn more but did not have time.

Shum (1992) described the then state of computerisation as the 'end of the beginning'. In the rest of this paper, we shall seek to describe insights that have been gained from the experience and the lessons that can be learned.

Table 1.1 Uptake of computers amongst GPs

Date	Uptake (%)	Source	Region
1986	5–10	Prescription for change	UK
1988	20	Brown et al.	Oxford
1989	45	Bradley and Watkins	UK
1992	76 in use + 10 on order	Shum	Surrey

Computerisation driven by Government legislation

The public sector in the UK has undergone a huge change from the mid-1980s onwards. A competitive ethos and the supplier/purchaser model has been introduced in all areas of local government and more recently in the NHS.

Generally, this degree of change was accompanied by an increase in IT support and this led to a number of characteristic problems which may be identified across different service areas. They are caused by the way that change is driven in the public sector. Change is driven by the introduction of legislation causing changes in information needs and working practices. In general, change is much more easily handled if introduced in an incremental fashion. However, legislative change often enforces revolutionary change at a time determined not by management but by political will.

Consider, for example, the provision of computers for administration of housing benefit. On April 1, 1988, new housing benefit regulations were brought in. Suppliers of software systems to local authorities were required to have new information systems in place and ready to go live on that date. At least one supplier was unable to deliver and this resulted in an untested bug-ridden code being released to customers. The resulting problems nearly bankrupted the supplier and caused major problems for local authorities (Gillies, 1992). Similar problems were reported at the implementation of the Community Charge (Gillies, 1990) and the Council Tax in 1993.

The imposition of new contracts in 1990 for GPs was equally traumatic. The requirements for information systems had been known since the 1986 Green Paper and the 1987 White Paper. Therefore, information systems were available. The introduction of these contracts acted as a stimulus to the use of computer systems. However, after three years, there was evidence that doctors had not yet assimilated their new tools fully (Shum, 1992; Chisholm and Gillies, 1994).

The methods and sources used

The evidence used in the study

The diversity of practice requires the investigator to draw on the widest possible base of reliable evidence, drawing on a range of sources to take account of regional, social, cultural and organisational diversity.

Historical data drawn from surveys

The most reliable national statistics are those provided by Government departments and agencies. Thus, where possible the study uses figures from the Department of Health (DoH) and the Office of Health Economics (OHE). However, these are not available for all years and, additionally, they do not reflect local variations and diversity which are characteristic of primary healthcare.

To take account of this, the study makes reference to regional surveys, principally Shum's study of GPs in East Surrey (Shum, 1992), Brown's study of GPs in the Oxford region (Brown, 1988), Hayes' study of practice in Sheffield (1985) and an early survey in Derbyshire (Madely and Metcalf, 1978).

Personal experience

The author has been involved with the computerisation process at first hand. He was the principal course leader during the training programme for Scottish GPs from 1989 to 1992. This involved working closely with the National Committee of Scottish GPs responsible for advising the Scottish Office on GPASS (General Practice Administrative System for Scotland), the system used by over 90% of the doctors who have computer systems in Scotland.

The author visited regions of Scotland (Strathclyde, Lothian, Tayside and Galloway) and trained in excess of 400 doctors and their staff. Training has also been carried out in England on behalf of a number of FHSAs.

Interviews

In order to gain specific detail and information regarding current experience, five practices were visited and in-depth interviews carried out in the North West of England. They were chosen to provide maximum variety in terms of size, location and management style. The information collected from these interviews may not be generalised but is useful to show the diversity of experience amongst doctors. The five practices were as follows:

Practice 1   A one-doctor practice in a medium size town (population, 30 000) with a small patient list, and a young doctor with five years' experience of using computers, most of which was gained in a previous much larger practice.

Practice 2   A six-doctor fundholding practice located in a health centre in the middle of a town on the eastern edge of the Greater Manchester conurbation. The doctors had a diverse range of experience and attitudes towards the computer. The practice had had a computer for five years.

Practice 3   A three-doctor inner-city practice in Greater Manchester with 5000 patients, a branch surgery and two years' experience with a computer system.

Practice 4   A single-doctor suburban practice with seven years' computer experience which formed part of a larger health centre serving a total of 13 000 patients.

Practice 5   A one-doctor inner-city practice with no computer experience and a similar number of patients to the first practice.

All interviews were carried out during 1993, all except practice 1 in the first half of the year.

Observations

Comparison of implementation in Scotland, and the rest of mainland Britain

In general, because of differing political patterns in Scotland, and the rest of mainland Britain, the process of commercialisation within the NHS has met with different reactions. In England and Wales, it has been accepted, often with resignation by the doctors and health administrators. In Scotland, it has been resisted as far as is possible within legal constraints. This has led to a much more centralised and co-operative approach to healthcare provision in Scotland (Gillies, 1993).

In England and Wales, the whole organisational structure has become more fragmented with more independent fundholding GPs, and rapid adoption of trust status by the majority of hospitals and supplying organisations. This has provided an opportunity for private sector software suppliers to sell their products in a commercial marketplace. It has also made it difficult for centralised strategies and solutions to be provided. However, the culture prevalent in England and Wales, and the ambiguous relationships between many doctors and the FHSAs, would make such an imposed standard solution unacceptable in many cases. The dominant feature in this approach has been competition.

By contrast, in Scotland, the process has been driven by the RHBs, which have provided free software for practices, thus ensuring that over 90% of those practices which are computerised use the same (GPASS) system. The majority of Scottish doctors have welcomed this in a spirit of co-operation rather than regarded it as a controlling mechanism. However, it may be argued that it restricts competition and choice and as such runs contrary to the spirit of the Government's reforms. In Scotland, where the Government enjoys very limited political support this is not a problem and may even be a favourable factor.

The effects

The first and obvious difference has been in the costs of the systems to the practices. In England and Wales, the doctors have borne the cost of the systems, although the new contract does provide for a 50% refund of those expenses construed as running costs. In Scotland, the software is free and the hardware is available at a 50% discount.

There is no doubt that the commercial systems provided in England have been more advanced technologically than the Scottish GPASS system over the period of the last five years. Driven by the need to achieve competitive advantage, the commercial suppliers have supplied highly sophisticated multi-user systems. The superior technical merit was illustrated by a disastrous attempt to introduce a particularly poor version of GPASS into the commercial English market without the benefits of the support provided in Scotland.

The benefits of the collective approach are less obvious and less glamorous. Most arise simply from the fact that the vast majority of GPs use the same system. For example, when the health board wishes to collect information on prescribing patterns they receive data in one format. At a meeting of English medical advisers, the author collected 19 different data formats that they encountered in their work.

The benefits of the Scottish system help both the doctors and the health boards. The health board is able to supply basic patient data (name, address, sex, DOB, etc.) for any practice implementing GPASS for the first time. If this central provision of data saves one minute per patient, then in a 10 000 patient six-doctor practice it will save nearly 20 working days of effort. In the longer term, compatibility makes checking for discrepancies between doctors' records and information held by the board much simpler. This has both financial and healthcare benefits.

Compatibility also allows much greater provision for training; user groups and technical support leading to greater knowledge at lower cost. The system is attractive because it originates from a doctor (a *Scottish* doctor) and the development programme has continued to be strongly influenced by input from doctors through local groups and a national committee. This has led to greater identification and ownership of the system amongst the GP community.

These benefits notwithstanding, some Scottish doctors have expressed the view that the centralised approach has meant that the GPASS software is inferior to its commercial counterparts.

However, the commercial packages are not without their problems. The various data formats, all incompatible for reasons of commercial exclusivity, make it difficult for doctors to extract data for audit and analysis purposes. They also cause worry when a commercial supplier appears to be in financial difficulties, as happened to a major player in 1992.

There are also some basic errors in some systems. The suppliers range from large commercial concerns to systems supplied by an individual who wrote a system for his friend who was a doctor and then thought of further market potential.

There are some basic problems which arise from poor systems thinking and design. For example, under the new contractual arrangements, those doctors who have assumed control of their own budgets, known as 'fundholders' have additional information requirements compared with their colleagues. Most suppliers of information systems can provide an add-on module to cater for this need. However, the degree of integration of these extra functions is variable.

Practices 1 and 2 in the interviews both used the same system. In practice 1, which is under the budgetary control of the local FHSA, the system is favoured by the doctor for its ease of use. It avoids the use of coding by allowing doctors to select diagnoses from menus. This encourages standardisation as well as being easy to learn.

However, in the fundholding practice (practice 2), the system is less easy to use. The fundholding module is in practical terms a separate system, which requires much of the clinical data held on the main system to be re-entered into the fundholding module. Thus, the author talked to a typist whose sole job was to re-enter data from a print-out from the main patient records system into the fundholding module. No facility existed for integration of data or even electronic transfer of files *en bloc*.

Work from other disciplines has highlighted the importance of correct implementation as a more significant factor than the technical merit of the software (Gillies and Baugh, 1993). Further, software that reinforces unhelpful working practices such as the above is likely to prove disastrous in the longer term.

Individual experiences of doctors within the North West of England

Practice 1: One-doctor, 1200 patients, non-fundholder

This practice had a well-established computer system and the doctor and his practice manager were very comfortable with the technology. Extensive use of the computer system was made for preventive medicine through screening and immunisation programmes. The system used was a multi-user system with terminals in the reception area, consulting room and practice manager's office. System maintenance and housekeeping was carried out by the practice manager, although the doctor was obviously highly computer literate. The system was used for all patient records, prescribing, screening and compiling practice reports. Discussions were currently underway about direct links to the FHSA for reporting purposes. Confidentiality issues were a high priority and a mailbox system was under discussion to prevent the FHSA from having general access to the system.

The biggest problem highlighted was the transfer from manual to computer patient records. Apart from the issue of the amount of time involved, the quality of information was considered critical. 33% of paper-based records showed inconsistencies, for example members of the same household were listed as living at different addresses. As a result, the input of patient data was handled by the doctor himself, in order to preserve the integrity of the data as far as possible.

Practice 2: Six-doctor, 9000 patients, fundholder
This large practice showed some of the problems of trying to establish computer usage amongst a diverse group of professionals. In theory, all six doctors used the system. However, there was significant reluctance amongst the two oldest doctors (both over 50 years of age) in the practice. This meant that there was inconsistency in the manner in which the computer system was used. Four of the doctors used terminals in their consulting rooms to record information from consultations directly onto the system. The remaining doctors did not have direct contact with the system but recorded all details on paper and then passed their paper records to the reception staff for them to record on the computer system.

The consequences of this for data integrity are potentially serious with an extra person in the data entry chain. Errors may arise from either accidental mis-transcription or misinterpretation arising from a lack of clinical expertise.

The author found a lack of clarity in the line of responsibility for the computer system between the practice manager and the doctor who was regarded as the most computer literate by her colleagues. For example, when the practice manager was asked who the data protection officer was, he stated that he was. He later rang to correct this information as it transpired that the doctor was in fact the registered person.

This was a fundholding practice but the information required for managing the budget was dealt with almost entirely separately. This was partly a consequence of the design of the information system. As a result, much data was printed out from the main clinical system and re-entered into the fundholding module. The implications of this were a good deal of wasted effort and major doubts about the integrity of the data.

This practice had the appearance of being comfortable with the technology but on closer examination had some major problems. Currently these are being addressed through a considerable investment in administrative staff, but in the longer term there are serious implications for the fundamental integrity of their information.

Practice 3: Three-doctor practice, 5000 patients, non-fundholder
This inner city practice had a computer system based around a single machine. Many of the characteristics of this practice arose from its inner city location.

- Due to high levels of crime in the area, it was felt that the computer could not be left in the surgery overnight. As a consequence the system was based upon a laptop machine shared by all the staff.
- The practice was characterised by a high level of patient and staff turnover.
- The use of a single laptop meant that staff had limited access to the computer. The absence of formal training for staff arriving since the adoption of the system in 1991 had compounded this inexperience and led to a considerable lack of confidence amongst the administrative staff in the use of the computer. This problem was made worse by the existence of a branch surgery where all data was recorded on paper, transferred physically to the main surgery and then entered onto the computer.

These factors led to very limited use of the computer system and a dependence upon the FHSA for certain information, e.g. the FHSA supplied the list of the women to be called for cervical screening. Experience elsewhere suggests that this dependence is undesirable unless there are strong links between the doctor's own computer systems and the FHSA. This was clearly not the case here.

The system was also not used for compiling the practice report, which again causes duplication of work and introduces the possibility of data transcription errors.

The personnel interviewed, both the doctor and his staff, felt that these problems were exacerbated by poor documentation, poor training and unnecessary complexity of the computer processes.

Practice 4: One-doctor, part of 13 000 patient health centre, non-fundholding
This practice had had a computer system for the last seven years. It was shortly to be replaced by a system which is linked directly to the FHSA. The experience gained has led to clearly defined division of tasks amongst the various staff, with much of the routine information (e.g. registration, patient record updates, health screening) entered not by GPs but by the administrative staff. The GP had responsibility where clinical factors are paramount (e.g. prescriptions, medication, family planning).

When the new system is installed, direct links to the FHSA will permit many tasks, e.g. patient registration and screening details to be handled directly by the FHSA without compromising the integrity of the data.

This practice appeared relatively comfortable with the technology. This is attributable to the length of time that a system has been in place. The doctor and staff in this practice reported the same paucity of documentation and training as the last practice, but have overcome problems gradually over the years. The location of this practice in a larger health centre was helpful through the pooling of knowledge and expertise with other doctors and staff in the same building.

Practice 5: One-doctor, 1200 patients, non-fundholding
This practice had no computer system. It had managed with a card-based system so far because of its small size. However, it has shortly to install a system which would be linked to the FHSA. The patient records and other data were kept on card indexes. The implications of this was that much more time was spent on filing and recording patient information than in Practice 1 which was comparable in size. More significant perhaps was the potential for error and the difficulty of spotting errors. Experience in other practices has revealed a discrepancy rate of 5 to 10% between paper recording systems and the FHSA's central records.

Issues identified

Evidence for traumatic change

Shum (1992) found that the usage of installed systems was well below the maximum potential levels (*see* Figure 1.4).

This was supported by the interviews which revealed in a few specific cases, a lack of practitioners' knowledge about their systems, problems in coding diagnoses and major cultural problems in practices where partners have often split into 'pro' and 'anti' computer camps. There is a cultural hurdle here because many GPs were not used to working together and effectively compromising their clinical judgements in order to reach a consensus. This can provide another very serious barrier to the successful implementation of the computer system.

It suggests that the global figures for computerisation cited earlier may not reflect the actual usage of systems. This failure to optimise use of the technology may be attributed to the failure to manage the process of change through an evolutionary process.

A further consequence is the worrying situation where a system is in use and apparently functioning correctly, but doctors and practice staff have insufficient knowledge to recognise a major potential lack of data integrity.

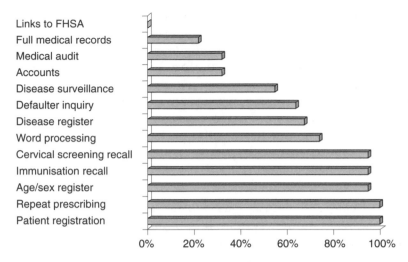

Figure 1.4 The utilisation of computers by 1992.
Source: Shum, 1992.

Did change have to be traumatic?

There is much evidence from studies of the introduction of computers in different types of organisations which indicates that revolutionary change is not the best way to achieve maximum benefit (Gillies and Baugh, 1993; Gillies and Smith, 1994). However, it might appear that the GP community was forced to embrace computers almost overnight in the light of the new 1990 contract and the associated information requirements.

However, this was not the case in reality. If one considers implementation as a process somewhere between the ideal case of gradual change and a 'big bang' approach then one can see that it has been possible to implement computer systems in an evolutionary way. Unlike the local government cases mentioned above, the information needs of GPs under the 1990 contract (DoH, 1989) could be foreseen in the earlier legislation (DoH, 1986, 1987) giving four years for software providers to prepare their systems and their clients.

Doctors were receptive to the need for better information. As far back as 1978, there was some recognition that good quality paper-based information systems were needed (*see* Table 1.2).

The two principal advantages of an evolutionary approach are a recognition of the need for planning and the opportunity to assimilate change in small doses.

An unusual feature of the computerisation of general practices is the ability to compare the implementation in different parts of the UK. Cultural, political and organisational differences between Scotland and the rest of mainland Britain provide a good basis for comparison, albeit in a qualitative manner.

Table 1.2 Percentage of doctors using a specific recording system to meet a particular need

Recording system	Use by doctors
Age/sex register	23.1%
Chronic sick register	12.8%
Hospital referrals log	7.5%
Diagnostic index	6%
Register of patients in hospital	4%

Source: Madely and Metcalfe, 1978.

Differences in implementing change

It has been noted above that evolutionary change is generally more advantageous than revolutionary change. A basic process of evolutionary change for GPs from a paper-based system to a computer-based system might be considered in terms of the following stages:

- make paper system computer-ready
- implement common diagnostic coding policy within the practice
- implement and evaluate pilot single-user system computerising only those functions which bring maximum benefits at minimum cost
- expand scope of single-user system to include all major functions
- implement multi-user system putting terminals on doctors' desks.

All practices would benefit from the use of a single-user system as a pilot implementation. The advantage of using a single-user system as an intermediate step is that it reduces the initial problems of computerisation to more manageable proportions. It allows diagnostic coding practice to be established and if restricted initially to certain areas (e.g. screening and repeat prescribing) it can provide rapid benefits at limited cost. Any further implementation will reflect the law of diminishing returns.

It allows the more sceptical members of the practice to be convinced before embarking upon wholesale change.

Some practices never progress beyond this point. Their reasons are not all bad:

- in small practices, a multi-user system may be unnecessary
- computerising patient records beyond limited areas may be expensive and time-consuming and unjustified by benefits
- the practice may not be able to support the extra technical expertise to run a multi-user system in an environment such as UNIX
- the practice may regard the presence of a computer terminal in a consulting room as an unwarranted intrusion upon doctor-patient consultations
- a limited solution which works well may be more effective than a more ambitious solution which fails.

Most Scottish practices went through this experience simply because GPASS was not offered as a multi-user system at first. Many have now progressed to multi-user systems, having benefited from the experience of using the simpler system first.

They have often found moving from single-user DOS-based GPASS to multi-user UNIX-based GPASS a bigger step than computerisation itself. The problem of establishing and running a computer network in a non-technical environment is often underplayed by suppliers keen to sell their products. In many cases it results in either the practice managers spending large amounts of time acting as *de facto* IT manager, or the recruitment of a specific IT manager, which must be justified in terms of benefits to the practice.

In England and Wales, most systems were implemented as multi-user solutions. Shum's survey (1992) suggests that many are still struggling to assimilate the level of change required and that usage has not progressed far beyond what would normally be achieved with a smaller pilot implementation.

The problem of coding

One of the fundamental problems of any information system whether paper- or computer-based is the problem of diagnostic coding. Computerisation does not create this problem but does highlight it. Problems of coding may be considered under three headings:

- the basic problem
- the coding schemes themselves
- implementation of coding.

The basic problem

The basic problem of coding is that the aim is to describe a fuzzy problem (diagnosis) in terms of a discretely structured classification system. The result is that the coding process itself must be imprecise and subjective. As such, there is scope for disagreement amongst colleagues as to what is the correct code for a given diagnosis.

Since computer systems do not understand medicine but merely match alphanumeric strings it is essential that the codes are entered consistently. Further, if externally derived search routines are used, the codes must be defined in the manner expected by the search routine. The ultimate consequences of incorrect coding are the incorrect recording of diagnoses leading to incorrect information submitted to external bodies. Procedures for avoiding some of these problems are described below under implementation of coding.

The coding schemes themselves

The nature of the coding schemes themselves can cause problems. In order to compile a hierarchical scheme to cover the whole of medicine, it is necessary to define a huge number of individual codes. Since it is not practical to define such a scheme from scratch, it is inevitable that the process is one of collation rather than creation. For example, schemes such as the Read Code Classification are based upon a collection of schemes from other sources.

This produces some interesting quirks. For example, under Read, there are many codes derived from an American medico-legal scheme. Thus a GP can classify your complaint readily as judicial execution or assassination in an opera house. However, coding for common complaints is complicated by a bewildering range of apparently similar options, e.g. asthma, history of asthma, family history of asthma.

The second problem can arise in searching for a suitable code. With a hierarchical scheme such as Read, it is possible to provide a tree-like search facility homing in on the exact code required to the desired level of detail. A difficulty arises sometimes when a logical search path appears to take a sharp bend leaving you where the originator of the coding scheme feels you should be rather than where you feel you ought to be.

Implementation of coding
In order to minimise the difficulties of coding, it is highly desirable that the partners in a practice establish a strategy for coding amongst themselves. The issues to be resolved include:

• Will all the patient records be coded?
• If not, which group of patients and what conditions?
• What level of detail is required?
• What codes will be used for standard conditions, e.g. asthma, abnormal smears?
• Should coding be carried out at the time of the consultation or retrospectively?
• How much of the historical data should be coded?

One of the particular pitfalls of a single-user system is that data entry is often carried out by a non-medical person. Instances have been recorded where the doctors provide the data entry person with a clinical diagnosis recorded as a text description, e.g. asthma, and they are left to translate this imprecise text description into a code. This amounts to asking them to make a clinical judgement for which they have no expertise.

Security and integrity issues

One of the prime concerns of doctors is patient confidentiality. This is one area where there are clear benefits of a multi-user system where basic security features such as password protection and user identification codes are standard. Whilst it is possible to protect an application running in single-user mode under DOS, the operating system itself is not designed with security in mind and it is always possible that a determined hacker could override security that is local to the application.

More alarming is the ignorance of many practices about their legal requirements. An audit carried out by the IT manager of one FHSA found that over 90% of practices had inadequate entries under the Data Protection Act, leaving themselves open to prosecution.

In a professional community where ethics and confidentiality have always had the highest priority it is essential that computerisation does not compromise standards through ignorance. Where there is a lack of computer knowledge amongst staff, specific instances clearly show ignorance of the consequences for data accuracy and confidentiality.

Training and documentation

This article has already highlighted the problem of under-utilisation of the system functionality. The interviews carried out highlighted the following as barriers to greater use in specific cases:

- poor initial training
- poor documentation
- lack of time and support for ongoing development of skills.

Training was typically supplied free at the time of purchase. However, typically this took place over two days for the whole practice. This creates a number of issues. First, staff start at a very low knowledge level and cannot possibly gain maximum benefit from a concentrated block of time at the very start. When involved in training activities with similar staff, the author teaches in day or half-day blocks separated by a four to six week assimilation period.

The second issue is that different staff have different needs and may not receive the best training when working together. The author has witnessed the spectacle of doctors working with their administrative staff happily on a training course until a sentence or phrase requires typing. At that point some doctors will sit back, hand the keyboard to their staff member, and say 'Oh, typing, that's your job!' unwilling to reveal their one finger data entry style amongst a group of administrative staff.

The third training issue is that of ongoing training. There is a need for further training as the user progresses from a novice to an advanced user. The general view that this cannot be afforded, either in time or money, fails to take account of the opportunity cost of under-used facilities and the time spent trying to determine how to do a specific task.

Good training does exist. However, it is not always available from the suppliers of proprietary software systems. For independent suppliers of training, the fragmented commercial marketplace outside Scotland makes the provision of high-quality training awkward and expensive. By contrast, the centralised approach adopted in Scotland meant that it was possible to provide a training programme based upon good practice at an economical rate.

The quality of documentation is generally lamentable. It tends to be written by a computer literate person who fails to take account of the target audience. Even where professional writers are brought in to produce the manuals, they do not generally have a medical background and do not appreciate the perspective of the average reader. Unfortunately, this is a widespread problem through the software supply industry and is not unique to medicine.

An interesting exception to this rule is the documentation supplied with the public domain epidemiology software, Epi Info, which is of a high standard. This is a public domain product, which offers better documentation than some expensive commercial products (Gillies, 1994).

Conclusions

The current state of computerisation in primary healthcare in the UK is of much technology in place, but that few practices are making full use of what is available. Some of the reasons for this have been explored. Although most surgeries now have systems in place, many of the problem areas could yet be addressed to advantage. The author recommends the following prescription for current ills:

- considerable investment in documentation and training, either by the doctors themselves or by the FHSAs
- assistance for the profession from IT professionals on the management of systems
- recognition by IT professionals of the specific needs of the doctors
- the need for strategies and guidelines to facilitate data communication and exchange in a fragmented marketplace.

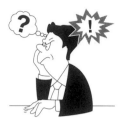

Questions to think about

Consider the articles above and ask yourself the following questions:

1 How far did the wave of reforms around 1990 deliver an information infrastructure in line with the stated policy of the day?
2 What were the major barriers to a successful implementation?
3 What are the legacies of the situation described here for today's PCG(T)s?
4 What benefits have we inherited for today's PCG(T)s?

The legacy

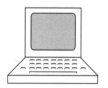

On-line resource
Visit the GPASS Evaluation Project website accessible in the Chapter 1 section of the website. You may like to compare this with the PRIMIS (Primary Care Information Services) project dealt with in Chapter 3, whose website is accessible from that section.

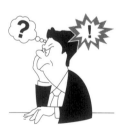

Questions to think about

Consider the information available from the GPASS evaluation project and ask yourself the following questions:

1 How far would the Scottish infrastructure currently meet the needs of English PCG(T)s?
2 How far would the future plans detailed on the site meet the needs of English PCG(T)s?
3 With the benefit of hindsight were the views expressed in the publications above justified?

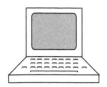

On-line resources
To complete this chapter read the respective English and Scottish information strategy documents, *Information for Health* and *Taking Action,* available on-line through the Chapter 1 section of the website accompanying this book.

 Key points

By the end of this section, you should be able to:

1 Identify the different development paths taken in England and Scotland.
2 Identify the strengths and weaknesses of each system.
3 Understand how we have arrived at the situation we have today.
4 Analyse whether the predictions made in 1993 and 1995 by the author have proved correct.

2

Primary care information systems

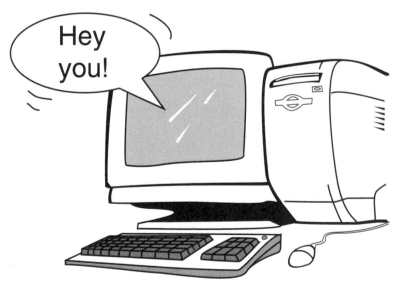

'I know I'm supposed to be a PATIENT record system
but how much longer are you going to be?'

Introduction

In this chapter, we shall consider primary care information systems by considering the rules for accreditation for general practice systems. We shall consider their content, scope and effectiveness.

What are the rules for accreditation?

The following notes are taken from the Introduction to RFA99:

Requirements for Accreditation (RFA) was first introduced in April 1993 to ensure General Medical Practice computer systems provided an agreed core functionality and conformed to national standards. RFA99 supersedes RFA version 4 (RFA4) published in June 1997.

It is considered important that GP computer systems are accredited to RFA. FHSL(97)47, issued on 8 December 1997, strongly recommended that health authorities should only reimburse GP expenditure in respect of new systems, changes of supplier or major upgrades to existing systems if the expenditure related to a system accredited to RFA4. It is expected that this guidance will be updated to reflect the position of RFA99 as the new minimum standard for general practice computer systems.

Information for Health

The Primary Care – Requirements for Accreditation Steering Group approved the start of work on RFA99 in September 1998, at the time *Information for Health* (the Strategy) was published. Since further guidance and clarification were needed before the more wide-ranging changes arising from the Strategy could be considered, it was decided that the main purpose of RFA99 should be to refine and clarify existing functional requirements already present in RFA4. This would ensure that all requirements are clear, relevant and up to date, and that they can be measured objectively. However, there are a small number of important new additions, including MIQUEST (Morbidity Information QUery Export SynTax) and PRODIGY, and for the first time, RFA99 includes some requirements for training.

RFA99 has also been produced against the background of the new Purpose and Scope for RFA, which was agreed by the Steering Group in April 1998 and endorsed by the NHS Executive. This is included in the Strategic Statement part of this document.

As a consequence, RFA99 provides a firm basis on which future requirements for GP systems can be built.

Development of RFA99   In order to ensure that RFA99 meets the requirements of the key stakeholders, a series of working groups were established to review RFA4 and make recommendations for RFA99. Each group had a representative of the GP profession, the NHS executive, a health authority and a supplier.

Purpose   RFA99 is a technical document for suppliers to develop systems for testing and accreditation. It will also be of use to health authorities and purchasers of GP systems by providing guaranteed levels of functionality where accredited systems are being purchased. A number of other documents are referenced which may be obtained through the NHS Information Authority Helpline on 0121 625 2711. The majority are also available on the CD-ROM version of RFA99.

Not all the functions specified in this document are mandatory. Optional requirements are clearly indicated as such. However, where these facilities are offered they must meet the relevant specification.

Scope and content   RFA99 has been restructured into a more logical sequence, and a glossary has been added. It now consists of the following parts:

Part CR   Core requirements and services
Part ST   Supplier services: support and training
Part GF   General functionality
Part MI   Messaging and information exchange
Part KR   Knowledge related functionality
Part SS   Strategic statement
Annex 1   Accreditation flow chart
Annex 2   Required documentation
Glossary

Part CR: Core requirements and services   This is a new part which draws together and updates general aspects of services and requirements that impact on, or underlie, other parts of RFA. It includes privacy and security, Year 2000 conformance, Read codes, NHS number, data standards and system configuration.

Part ST: Supplier services: support and training   This is a new part which updates previous requirements on support and introduces new requirements on documentation and training. It recognizes the need for practices to work in partnership with suppliers to benefit from the training offered.

Part GF: General functionality   This part updates previous RFA requirements on practice and patient administration, prescribing and reporting facilities.

Requirements for accreditation introduction

Part MI: Messaging and information exchange   This part sets out requirements on the connection of GP systems to NHSnet for the exchange of EDI and e-mail messages between GP systems and NHS organisations. It specifies the HA/GP and clinical messages for which testing is available, and sets out the status of each message for accreditation purposes. This part has been completely rewritten to make the relationships between the different documents it references clear.

Part KR: Knowledge related functionality   This is a new part which introduces requirements for MIQUEST and PRODIGY. The detailed specifications for these are not contained within this document, but are available separately.

Part SS: Strategic statement   The purpose of this section is to provide suppliers with an indication of other IT initiatives and projects which may be included in future versions of RFA.

Implementation guidance notes   RFA4 introduced the concept of implementation guidance notes (IGNs). These are issued from time to time to clarify specific sections of RFA, explain how it relates to other initiatives, provide additional information and so on. Their purpose is primarily to assist suppliers in their development work, but they will also be of interest to other recipients of RFA as they help to explain the implications of implementing RFA and investing in RFA accredited systems. It is expected that IGNs will be issued for RFA99. All RFA4 IGNs have been absorbed into RFA99.

Conformance testing   Conformance testing is a prerequisite for accreditation and will be carried out by the NHS Information Authority. Suppliers will be expected to sign a contract with the authority for testing; this will include a service level agreement for the testing process.

The core requirements and general functionality parts of RFA99 continue to provide details of test conditions; these are intended as examples to give suppliers an indication of what will apply in the testing process. However, it would be inadvisable for suppliers to base their system development solely on the examples of the test conditions outlined in these parts.

Testing will also be dependent upon a declaration of preparedness by the supplier and the satisfactory completion of a number of preconformance tests. **Annex 2** lists the documents which must be produced as part of the testing process.

The NHS Information Authority will have control of the testing process and if products are deemed to be incomplete or ill prepared testing will be suspended. Full details of the procedures for testing and accreditation are contained in **Annex 1**.

Clear now? In simple terms, the RFA tells us what a GP system should contain. It is unlikely that any practice would obtain reimbursement for a system without RFA approval these days. If you are still unsure try reading Chapter 2 of *Information and IT for Primary Care* (although at the time of writing, RFA4 was the latest version: that's the one before RFA99, don't ask!)

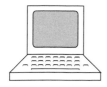

On-line resource
Now read the rest of the RFA99 document accessible from the Chapter 2 section of the website. It is available in Acrobat format, so you can download each section and read it off-line. At the time of writing, RFA2001 is being published. See the website for an update.

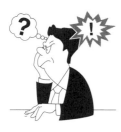

Questions to think about

Consider the RFA99 document, or RFA2001 if this is the latest version by the time you read this, and ask yourself the following questions:

1   How far does the information specified meet the needs of primary care?
2   What else do you want from a system?
3   How far can we control the efficacy of systems through the use of rules for accreditation?
4   If, when purchasing a new system, you are offered two RFA99 compliant systems, how are you going to choose between them, and why?
5   Which aspects of system design do you feel are tightly specified and which are only specified vaguely?
6   Do you think that RFA has provided a good means of ensuring that system suppliers meet the needs of their customers?

Acquiring a system

If you are involved in acquiring a system, you will find the following book very useful:

Shaw NT (2001) *Going Paperless: a guide to computerisation in general practice.* Radcliffe Medical Press, Oxford.

It may be ordered on-line via the Chapter 2 section of the website.

🔑 Key points

By the end of this section, you should be able to:

1 Discuss the contents of RFA99.
2 Discuss the merits and de-merits of rules for accreditation schemes.

3

Coding

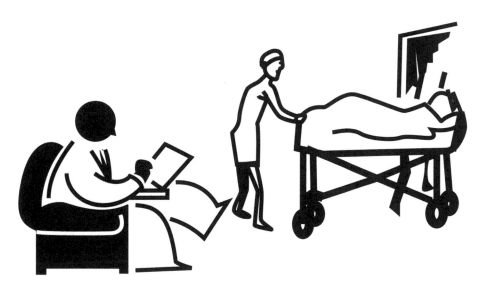

'I wish that there weren't so many letters in myocardial infarction.'

Introduction

In this chapter, we shall consider the use of coding systems in clinical systems. We shall focus upon Read codes as the commonest scheme in use in primary and community care, and the scheme specified in RFA99.

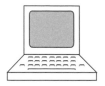

On-line resource
The NHS is committed to replacing the existing version of Read with a harmonised Read/SNOMED system. On the website, you will find the latest news on this development.

Read codes

Read codes are probably the second most important thing to get right about your information solution for your practice and primary care organisation (PCO); the first being the people. It is necessary to explain why coding is important and why Read codes are the only viable codes to use for your PCO. It is perhaps too much to hope that you should ever come to love Read codes, and frankly if you do, then the best advice is either to 'get a life' or seek professional counselling.

People use natural language to communicate and to describe things. It has the advantage of being known to everyone, is very flexible, and able to express shades of opinion and fuzziness. However, from the computer's point of view it is complex, inconsistent and requires a great deal of contextual information to interpret ambiguities. As we have seen, computers can process information quickly, but only if it is clear and unambiguous.

Just as human language has evolved to meet our information processing needs, so systems have evolved to meet the information processing needs of computers. Coding systems meet a need to describe the world of healthcare in concise and unambiguous ways.

The first major coding systems were used to describe diseases within epidemiology. Schemes of this type are ICD-9 and ICD-10. They provide a code made up of letters and numbers for just about every disease on the planet. They form a kind of Esperanto for epidemiologists. But disease coding is inadequate for primary care. Read codes are designed to cover the entire scope of primary healthcare.

First, let us consider five reasons why coding is essential, and second, why Read codes are the only suitable coding systems for PCOs.

Five reasons why coding is essential

1 Codes provide unambiguous information suitable for computer processing.
2 Codes allow standard morbidity data to be collected across a PCO population.
3 Codes allow the definition and implementation of standard clinical guidelines and protocols across the practices of a PCO.
4 Codes allow the collection of standard datasets for performance monitoring and clinical governance.
5 Coding facilitates comparison between and within PCOs.

Five reasons why Read codes are essential

1 Read codes cover the whole remit of primary care and much beyond primary care. My favourite is 'accidental poisoning occurring in an opera house'.
2 Read codes are hierarchical, allowing different levels of detail in different situations.
3 Read codes are updated every three months (drugs every month).
4 Read codes can be cross-referenced to all other major systems, e.g. ICD, OPCS, BNF, ATC, etc.
5 Coding only works if everyone talks the same language, Read codes are the UK NHS standard, therefore all other reasons are redundant.

In practice, the Read codes are intended to cover the following areas:

- diseases
- occupations
- history/symptoms
- examinations/signs
- diagnostic procedures
- radiology/diagnostic imaging
- preventive procedures
- operative procedures
- other therapeutic procedures
- administration
- drugs/appliances.

So, for the uninitiated, what do Read codes look like? They are generally described as being 'hierarchical' in nature. This means that the more letters or numbers you add the more precise the code becomes. Consider, for example, ischaemic heart disease. We shall use version 2 to illustrate, because it is still the most commonly used form of Read codes. In 'Read code speak', a simple letter 'G' represents the circulatory system. Add a '3' to make a 'G3' code and we get to a code for ischaemic heart disease. Add more numbers and we get more detail. If we carry on adding more numbers to our example it goes as follows:

An example of the use of Read coding

Circulatory system	G
Ischaemic heart disease	G3
Acute myocardial infarction	G30
Anterior acute myocardial infarction	G301
Acute anteroseptal myocardial infarction	G3011

These may look pretty daunting but there are important things that make Read codes less intimidating.

First, Read codes include 'synonyms' for clinical terminology. Thus within the coding system, whilst each concept has a preferred term, many also have synonymous terms. In our case, for example, 'G30 . .' represents 'acute myocardial infarction' which is known as the preferred term, but this concept may also be described as 'heart attack', 'acute MI', or 'MI' (among others). These terms are provided as synonyms and all have the same code as 'acute myocardial infarction' (G30 . .).

Second, much of the Read code terminology, once defined, can be hidden inside the computer system. Thus the system will automatically enter a G30 code when a doctor pulls any of the above terms off a list of clinical diagnoses on his or her computer screen.

In order to facilitate information sharing within a PCO, it is essential that coding policy is agreed at PCO level. The really important issue for PCOs is to set up all the practice information systems within their group to do the following:

What you need to do

1 Agree priority areas for coding across the PCO.
2 Agree what will be coded as a minimum for all practices across the PCO.
3 Agree to what level of detail information will be coded.
4 Agree standard codes across the PCO for all the information to be coded.

Fortunately, you don't have to make all these decisions on your own. There is a national project set up to assist with the collection of health data in general practice (hence its former name, CHDGP). The project has recently metamorphosed into the PRIMIS project.

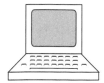

On-line resource
The PRIMIS project has a website accessible from the Chapter 3 section of the website accompanying this book. This has many useful resources including a very useful document known as the *Co-ordinators Handbook.*

For example, the *Co-ordinators Handbook* will tell you that the national project is focused around morbidity data in six key areas, linked closely to national health promotion targets:

• heart disease and related conditions
• cerebrovascular disease and related conditions
• hypertension
• diabetes
• asthma
• severe mental illness (psychoses and similar conditions).

The handbook provides guidelines which should form the basis of any PCO data collection initiative.

PRIMIS Guidelines for data collection

1   Whenever a patient presents with a morbidity (or morbidities) from the core data set, a recording of the appropriate code or codes is made to denote this encounter. The words appropriate code (or codes) refer to the morbidity; if other investigations are made which are referred to in the core data set, these are also to be recorded.
2   The relevant risk factors will also be recorded, again as appropriate.
3   Any numerical values associated with the code, such as blood pressure (BP) readings, should also be recorded.
4   The entry should be dated with the date on which the encounter took place.
5   The entry should be attributed to the clinician with whom the encounter took place.
6   The nature of the episode of the morbidity to which the encounter relates should be recorded.

The handbook provides lots of useful advice on how to maximise the quality of the data and is proof that there really are useful resources to be had free from the Internet (providing you buy this book first to tell you where to look!).

Having established the coding policy for your PCO which details the codes to be collected and the manner in which they are to be collected, it is then necessary to collect the coded information from the constituent practices. There are two key types of barriers here, technical and professional.

The technical barriers are based on the fact that all the major GP computer systems are incompatible and will not talk to each other. This is a major reason why it was suggested earlier that your PCO should try to focus upon a limited number of systems.

The professional barriers relate to concerns over data protection and confidentiality. There are often very genuine concerns on the part of professionals about the sharing of sensitive personal clinical information.

MIQUEST

The proposed solution to these twin problems is MIQUEST. MIQUEST is the combination of a software tool to overcome the technical barriers and a set of procedural guidelines to allay fears over confidentiality.

The technical part of MIQUEST is a query language and an interpreter. The query language is, funnily enough, a language in which you write queries. An example of a query would be 'How many patients have had a heart attack in the last year?'. Schematically we can think of MIQUEST as follows:

1   A query is written in the MIQUEST query language asking 'How many heart attacks occurred amongst your patients between 01/01/98 and 31/12/98?'.
2   The MIQUEST interpreter is able to translate the query written in MIQUEST speak into EMIS speak or MEDITEL speak, or whatever form the GP system requires. This causes the GP system to search its patient records to find how many G30 Read codes are recorded with dates in 1998.
3   It then sends the number to the MIQUEST interpreter which produces a report saying there were 42 cases during 1998. Now, MIQUEST may not be able to come up with the answer to 'Life the Universe and Everything' (which, incidentally, is 42). However, it is at least an attempt to deal with data collection from incompatible systems.

The second part of MIQUEST is the MIQUEST data collection protocol. These protocols contain full data security and confidentiality safeguards.

Safeguards specified by MIQUEST protocols

Before a query is run, the practice has:

- the opportunity to scrutinise the query
- the necessity of authorising the query before it can be run
- the safeguard that an external enquirer, e.g. a data collection scheme, may not access any strong patient identifiers, such as names, addresses, full dates of birth, full postcode, etc.

After a query has been run, the practice has:

- the opportunity to scrutinise the response
- the necessity of authorising the response before it is released to the enquirer.

In practice, I think that MIQUEST is a technically complex solution brought about as a response to bad historical planning and the victory of ideology over common sense. This wouldn't matter if there weren't some unfortunate consequences for PCOs. The problems generally lie with the MIQUEST interpreter.

Potential problems for PCOs with MIQUEST

- Each system requires its own interpreter.
- The interpreters must be written by the suppliers.
- The PCO needs an interpreter for every type of system within its group.
- Early interpreters proved unreliable.
- Some companies have been lukewarm in their support for MIQUEST, especially in providing MIQUEST interpreters for older systems.

As noted in the last section, RFA99, the rules for accreditation of GP systems to which suppliers must conform if they wish to attract funding for GP systems, include MIQUEST compatibility as a requirement. However, this will not deal with older systems which are already in place. There is no incentive for suppliers to develop interpreters for these systems.

In cases such as these, it will be necessary for the PCO to write special queries to interrogate those systems which cannot be accessed by MIQUEST. These queries must be written with great care to ensure compatibility with the MIQUEST queries. To view a sample MIQUEST query, refer to *Information and IT for Primary Care* (Gillies, 1999a).

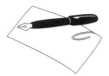

Practical activities

As a practical investigation into local IM&T plans, use the table below to identify the current coding policy of your organisation. If your own practice does no coding ask around the other members of your PCO to see what they are doing.

You may also like to investigate whether you have a local PRIMIS co-ordinator, who is a good person to get to know.

Clinical areas covered	Clinical terms identified	Read codes

Use the table below to identify what the coding policy of your organisation *should* be.

Clinical areas covered	Clinical terms identified	Read codes

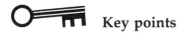 **Key points**

By the end of this section, you should be able to:

1 Describe what a Read code is.
2 Describe what a coding policy is.
3 Identify local policies in this area.

4

Information for health 1: the electronic health record

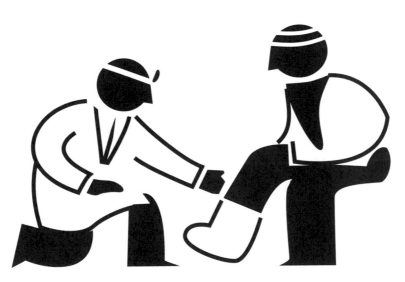

'I'm sorry your health record is empty . . .
I'll have to look you up in our illness records.'

Introduction

In this chapter we shall consider the concept and practicalities of the electronic health record (EHR).

The concept

At present, when a patient moves from one part of the NHS to another, their information moves with them in a very inefficient way. For example, when a patient moves their registration from one practice to another, even if their record exists in electronic form, it will almost certainly be printed out and then re-typed in at the next practice.

The concept of the EHR is that wherever the patient goes in the system, their record will follow electronically. It is an elegant concept, which is difficult to implement. The solution has a number of elements:

Elements of the EHR

- *A network to link every facility in the NHS.* This is the NHSnet. This is a technical matter for IM&T staff, and we shall leave it to them.
- *An agreed scope, language and syntax for the record.* This is the subject of a number of NHS projects on the electronic patient record (EPR).
- *An agreed way of recording data on the record.* The main issues here are concerned with coding, as explored in Chapter 3.
- *A way to keep the data within the record secure.* We shall look at our part in that and leave the rest to the IM&T staff.

Scope, language and syntax

In order to consider this topic, we must first review the work to date.

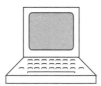

On-line resource

Read the following documents, available through the website accompanying this book:

- Chapter 2 of the *Information for Health* document
- The EPR section of the NHSIA website (Why isn't this the EHR section? Answers on a postcard to . . .)
- Integrated record keeping as an essential aspect of a primary care led health service (Rigby *et al.*, 1998).

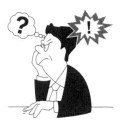

Questions to think about

Think about the following questions:

1 Why are EPRs and EHRs not even mentioned in the Scottish document *Taking action*?
2 Is there a useful distinction between EHRs and EPRs? How do you perceive it?
3 What are the limits of an EHR in terms of content? Should it include the following:
   • social care information
   • lifestyle information, e.g. smoking, drinking, sexual orientation, poverty index
   • Ethic origin?
4 Who should decide what is in a patient's EHR?
5 Who should be responsible for the accuracy of the EHR? – GP? Patient? Person entering data?

Security aspects of the EHR

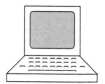

On-line resource
Read the following documents, available through the Chapter 4 section of the website accompanying this book:

• *Code of Connection to NHSnet for Full Service Access*
• *Confidentiality and Security Using NHSnet.*

The above resources will provide you with information on security aspects of the EHR.

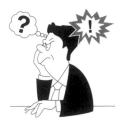

Questions to think about

1 Identify five distinctive threats to the security of your EHRs.
2 Identify a strategy for increasing security in respect of each threat.

Threat	Strategy for reducing risk

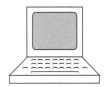

On-line resource
As a practical investigation, find the local implementation strategy (LIS) for your local area and see how it deals with the issues around the EHR. The Chapter 4 section of the website accompanying the book will direct you to LIS documents on the web.

Key points

By the end of this section, you should be able to:

1 Define and distinguish between EPRs and EHRs.
2 Understand the role of EHRs within the local and national information strategies.
3 Understand the benefits derived from the adoption of EHRs.
4 Understand the barriers to the adoption of EHRs.

5

Information for health 2: PCOs

Introduction

In this chapter we shall consider the implications of information policy as defined by the *New NHS White Paper* (DoH, 1997) and the *Information for Health* document for PCOs (DoH, 1998a).

The information needs of PCOs

To consider the information needs of PCOs, a traditional user requirements approach will be used. There are four stages:

- identify existing systems
- identify information requirements
- draw up logical design
- draw up physical design.

Identify existing systems

The venerable SSADM (Structured Systems Analysis and Design Methodology) tells us that the first stage of systems development is to identify existing systems. PCOs have inherited two types of system.

- *GP practice systems.* These systems exist in practices. They include both clinical and management information and have traditionally supported the clinical consultation and practice management function. The systems themselves vary from filing cabinets stuffed full of Lloyd George envelopes accompanied by card indexes and paper ledgers to modern integrated 32-bit Windows-based applications. As a general rule, the functions that have a positive effect on practice management and finances have been the most highly developed.
- *Health authority systems.* These systems have been held by the health authority and have been designed to ensure that such agencies could carry out their functions, including planning, ensuring that all patients have access to a GP and monitoring of practices.

Identify information requirements

To identify the information needs of the PCOs, we must go back before the *Information for Health* document to the 1997 White Paper to consider the six key tasks identified for PCOs:

Six key tasks for PCOs in the 1997 White Paper

- *Health commissioning.* To carry out effective health commissioning, PCOs need to match health needs of the population with health services provided by local hospitals and others. The health needs information comes from the GP clinical records. However, we also need information on the availability, cost and quality of services from the supply side of what we used to call the NHS internal market.
- *Health promotion.* To plan effective health promotion, we need to identify the health needs of the patients registered with the practices in our area. We also need to know what works. For this we need access to evidence and evidence-based resources such as clinical guidelines. The use of guidelines across the PCO should ensure consistent practice.
- *Monitoring performance* and *clinical governance.* Both activities are concerned with using information to monitor the quality and quantity of activities. As such, the information required is contained within the clinical records and prescribing and dispensing chapters of GP systems.
- *Resource deployment among general practice.* This is a PCO management function. However, the information required to assist in decision making is evidence both of health needs and practice activity. As such most of this can be drawn from the GP systems, the health needs coming from the patient records, and the activity data coming from the patient records and the prescribing and dispensing sections.

• *Work closely with other agencies.* Within the context of the new collaborative culture, it is necessary for PCOs to share information with other agencies both within the NHS and without.

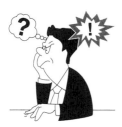

Questions to think about

The above activities depends on the PCOs having access to the information contained in the GP systems.

1 What barriers are there to this?

To help you, the table below divides potential barriers into technical, legal and human.

Type	Barriers
Technical	
Legal	
Human	

Draw up logical design

The logical design is a conceptual design. It shows what information is required, without specifying how these systems might be delivered in practice. From the information requirements, we may postulate the following as a logical design (*see* Figure 5.1).

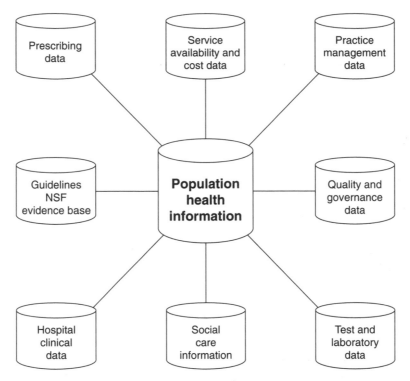

Figure 5.1 Schematic high level logical design.

In considering this design it is important to recognise that this is a logical design for a PCO system. It would also meet the needs of an individual practice system. The crucial difference is that PCOs need population-based information, which does not need to be, and should not be, identifiable. Practices on the other hand need patient-based information.

Patient information will be held in the clinical records in all the GP systems. PCOs need to be able to access this information in aggregated form for health commissioning, health promotion, performance monitoring and clinical govern-ance and epidemiological research. These purposes do not require identification of individual patients.

Many PCOs are starting to use tools such as MIQUEST to gather this data. MIQUEST has the advantage of building in the safeguards required to protect individual patient confidentiality.

For cross reference back to GP systems, a patient identifier may be added. This should be meaningless to the PCO, but allow GPs to identify their own patients where required.

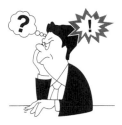

Questions to think about

1   In some cases we need to identify specific patients. What is the minimum data required to uniquely identify a patient?
2   In other cases, we need to prevent identification of specific patients. What is the minimum data that could enable a patient to be identified?

Draw up physical design

In considering the physical design of a system, we look at how the system might be organised in practice. The first stage is to identify which information is externally held and must be linked. The bottom row of the physical design is all information held externally. We shall consider some of the issues around this in the section, Inter-agency working.

For the remainder of the system, we may consider two options. The traditional approach is to link individual practice systems to a central hub system in the PCO (*see* Figure 5.2).

This approach maintains the integrity and autonomy of individual practices and their systems. It allows control of information passed from practices to PCOs, and allows the use of tools such as MIQUEST to extract only anonymous data from the practice systems to the centre.

The alternative is a single system for the PCO (*see* Figure 5.3).

In this design, the whole system runs from the PCO who would manage the system. External systems are linked to the central system. The controls and safeguards are provided at the point of access. Agreed protocols define rights of access for different staff. For example, patient-identifiable data would not be available to PCO staff. Your registered GP could be defined to have more complete access to your record than other clinicians. Doctors could have private areas where only they personally could have access.

The advantages of this system are:

- better data and coding integrity
- better management and potentially better security
- economies of scale
- ease of patient record movement between practices
- consistent application of standards and guidelines
- takes hassle of managing the IT system from the GPs.

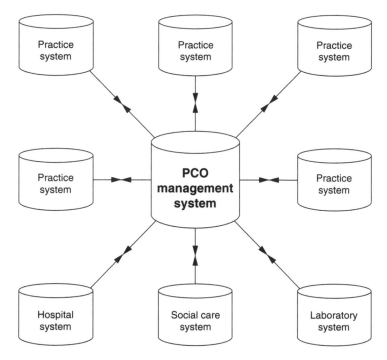

Figure 5.2 Traditional physical design.

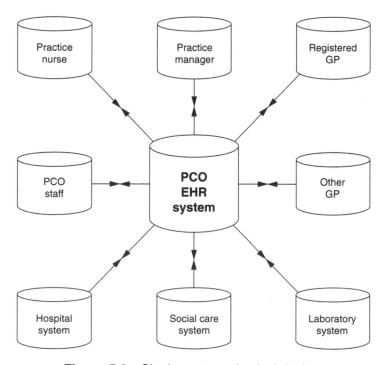

Figure 5.3 Single system physical design.

Against this are the disadvantages:

- threat to practice control and autonomy
- lack of ownership by clinicians and local staff
- removal of physical separation of patient and population-based data
- centralisation of data increases some risks.

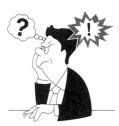 **Questions to think about**

1   How do you think the practices in your local area would react to a suggested system implementation of this type?
2   What would they state as their main objections?
3   Do you think these would be their real objections?

Inter-agency working

The final objective for PCOs is the need for PCOs to work with other non-NHS agencies. This will require the integration, or at least the exchange of information between the PCO and social services. This is not really a problem from a technical perspective.

The more significant problems are organisational and cultural. Studies by the author in the areas of mental health and childcare have revealed fundamental differences between the way that social care and healthcare organisations operate and the way they view information (*see* Table 5.1). Any PCO wishing to improve collaborative working with their local social care agencies must recognise these differences and take steps to negotiate compromises between agencies to take account of them.

We shall consider the implications of each in turn.

Coding

The coding of information is crucial to its effective management by computer-based information systems. Two key issues emerge in relation to coding in the inter-agency context. The first is the choice of coding systems. Within primary healthcare, the coding system now reaching universal acceptance is Read codes.

Table 5.1		
	What healthcare agencies do	*What social care agencies do*
Coding schemes	Read Codes, probably version 2	Incompatible local authority codes
Fundamental information entities	Patient-based health records	Family unit records
Attitudes to information collecting	More information is better	Only information leading to specific actions should be collected
Attitudes to confidentiality	Information may be shared amongst primary care team Information rarely stigmatises	Information should be tightly restricted Information can stigmatise

There appears to be little alternative to the use of Read codes as the basis of recording health data for inter-agency working. This will provide potential integration with the primary care electronic patient record (EPR). However, it is not likely that Read codes will be accepted readily by other agencies. Further it is unclear that Read codes can provide a universal coding standard for the information required to be contained within inter-agency working. One of the most helpful tools to assist joint working would be a mapping to convert key social care codes into Read codes.

Experience from the CHDGP data collection project suggests that the other major issue is the quality and consistency of coding. This is simply an extension of the issues discussed for intra-PCO working.

Fundamental information entities

Within any system, a crucial definition is the basic entity around which the system is built. Within an entity relationship model, the model is defined in terms of entities and the relationships between them. In most systems, either one entity is central or perhaps a system may be built around a relationship between two key entities, for example, library systems are defined by the relationship between borrowers and books (or other items). Clinical systems tend to be patient-focused; crucially information is linked to a single individual. This maps well onto the clinician–patient relationship and mode of working.

In social care, particularly in the context of children, the basic relationship is often with a family as a collective unit. This raises a number of issues. In data modelling terms, the issue becomes whether to model the family as a sub-entity of individual children or vice versa. As one family may have many children, it is more logical to use the family as the basic entity. However, this is then in conflict with the clinical perspective where information relates to an individual.

The PCO client will need to identify data held by social services about families with the specific individual children belonging to that family unit.

Attitudes to information collecting

In the healthcare sector, generally, there is a view that the more information collected the better, since this provides a richer picture of the health of the patient. Particularly in primary care, a wide range of factors may influence the health of the patient, and the immediate symptoms and stated reason for consulting the doctor may not be the most significant factors. This has sometimes had a negative influence on GP systems which have tended to become 'sinks' for information with little thought as to when the information may be retrieved and in what form.

By contrast, social workers tend to be much more minimalist in their information collection, preferring to emphasise that only relevant and targeted information, which is linked to specific courses of action, is collected. This has been explained in terms of the fear of litigation. This derives from cases where following a failure of care, it can be shown that information was available and not acted on.

The PCO may find the social care agencies less than grateful for a drip feed of inconclusive pieces of information relating to problems with children at risk or mental health patients housed in the community.

System usage must therefore be confined within agreed protocols, where it is clearly defined at what point action is required on the part of an individual professional or manager. However, it is recognized that even this may not be enough to 'sell' the system if a culture of fear exists.

Attitudes to confidentiality

Although health data is appropriately regarded as 'sensitive', the information in most child health records is not as sensitive as that relating to children being classified as 'at risk'. Much child health data is routine, for example recording the occurrence of childhood diseases. These data carry no stigma.

The very act of recording that a child may be at risk is extremely sensitive and changes the nature and context of all information regarding that child. For example, a child arriving at A&E with a fracture, with no history or label attached, is likely to receive only sympathetic treatment. The knowledge that this child has been deemed to be 'at risk' changes the nature of the information from a simple clinical diagnosis with consequences limited to treatment of the injury to potentially crucial evidence of significant abuse.

Thus, professional and parental attitudes to the information are likely to be fundamentally different. There is no significant need for excessive confidentiality over an incident such as a fracture arising from a genuine accident, unless there is a belief that the injury is caused by deliberate harm.

PCOs are increasingly likely to function as teams of practices operating themselves as teams. Thus, increasingly, healthcare is managed as a team activity. In most circumstances, it is professionally acceptable for all members of a team involved in the healthcare of a patient to have access to all relevant information.

However, the number of professionals involved in the process of care for a child deemed to be at risk may be considerable and the degree of their involvement may vary significantly. Therefore, it is appropriate to define a hierarchical model of access to sensitive information on a 'need to know' basis. For example, teachers and police officers may be involved in the process but need to have only partial knowledge. Within a school, there may be further differentiation between teachers designated to deal with child abuse cases, teachers with direct pastoral responsibility, such as form or year tutors, and class teachers.

This level of access may also apply to data input. In considering protocols, such as those suggested above, it may be appropriate to set different thresholds for action based on the specific training and experience of the person making the entry on the system. An alternative may be to restrict access to any information to facilitate human scrutiny by experienced and trained personnel of all reports made to the system.

Agreement over these issues, or indeed a lack of it, is likely to have a much greater impact on the working of the PCO in inter-agency working than technical limitations.

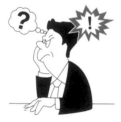

Questions to think about

A school nurse reports a child as showing unusual bruising and being unusually quiet. What needs to be done and who holds relevant information? Use the table below to consider this problem in terms of:

- Who should act?
- What should they do?
- What information do they need to act?
- Who holds that information?

Who should act?	What should they do?	What information do they need?	Who holds that information?

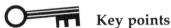 **Key points**

By the end of this section, you should be able to:

1 Understand the implications of the legislation for PCO information strategy.
2 Incorporate lessons from earlier units and modules into the information strategy.
3 Draw up an information strategy for your local PCO.
4 Provide guidance to your PCO on data collaboration with other agencies such as social services.

6

Information for health 3: patient information

Introduction

The *Information for Health* document places a new emphasis on information for patients. In this chapter, we shall consider the implications for information policy and some results. We shall visit websites aimed at patients.

Information and patients

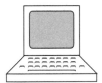

On-line resource
To consider this topic, read (or re-read) the following sections of key reports:

- Chapter 5 of *Information for Health*
- the Caldicott Report
- the discussion in the *BMJ* about NHS Direct.

To access these resources visit the Chapter 6 section of the website accompanying this book.

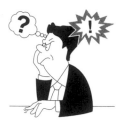

Questions to think about

1 Has NHS Direct delivered what was promised in *Information for Health*?
2 Do the safeguards to patients acting independently on advice from NHS Direct seem adequate?

On-line resources for patients

Visit three contrasting websites for patients.

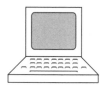

On-line resource
To consider the questions below, visit the three contrasting sites accessible from the Chapter 6 section of the website accompanying this book:

- Holland House Medical Centre: an award winning site from a local practice in Lytham St Annes
- NHS Direct
- CNN Health.

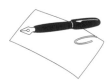

Practical activities

Compare the sites, thinking about the following questions:

- Which site is the most appealing?
- Which site loads most rapidly?
- Which site is the most understandable? (You may like to extract a section into Word and do a readability analysis)
- Which site provides the best advice on interpreting the information within? (You may like to extract a section into Word and do a readability analysis)
- Which site would you consult in a crisis and why?

You may like to use the table below to help you with your evaluation, rating each site according to the following scale:

1 very poor
2 poor
3 adequate
4 good
5 very good.

Criteria	Holland House	NHS Direct	CNN Health
Appeal			
Load time			
Ease of understanding			
Advice on interpretation			
Crisis management			

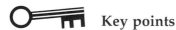 **Key points**

By the end of this section, you should be able to:

1 Find health information on the Web for patients.
2 Evaluate on-line sources.
3 Explain how and to what extent the NHS has implemented its stated goal of providing information for patients.
4 Understand the role of NHS Direct within the NHS.

7

Information for health 4: on-line resources

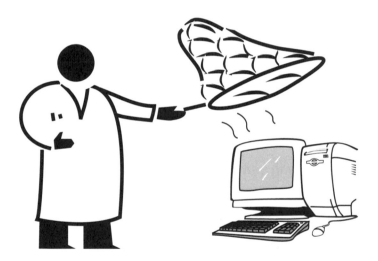

'Are you sure that the net is fine enough to keep out those virus thingies?'

Introduction

The combination of expansion in the Internet and a new emphasis on information resources has led to an increase in the resources available. In this chapter we shall tour the on-line resources for health professionals and evaluate their effectiveness and usefulness. As an introduction read the following unpublished paper from 1999.

The subservience of metaphor to technology and adaptability in the rapid growth of virtual health libraries on the World Wide Web (WWW)

Introduction

The 'virtual library' movement goes back to the origins of the World Wide Web (WWW) itself, and the founder of the Web, Tim Berner-Lee. Within the formal virtual library group, there are 14 sites dedicated to health issues (listed at http://vlib.org/Medicine.html). However, these are only one of a group of sites providing library-like resources on the Web. The largest group are those websites provided by physical libraries, of which the most famous is the National Library of Medicine in Washington.

Nearly all of these sites are characterised by the wide variety of resources available. However, many health professionals find them relatively unusable and often find themselves overwhelmed by the sheer amount of information available. Their problems are further exacerbated by doubts over the quality of the information provided.

In order to explore these issues, the author has returned to the first principles of interface design and considered the use of metaphor in the development of these virtual libraries, and how a richer metaphor may be used to improve the effectiveness of these sites.

Metaphor and the virtual libraries

The metaphor underpinning these virtual libraries is that of the document and that a library is made up of a collection of documents. Hence they all use a very simple interface and effectively provide a series of hyperlinks to documents stored locally and remotely. This brings a series of advantages, including simplicity, efficiency and practical consistency across a wide range of sites.

The disadvantage of this approach is the poverty of the metaphor employed. Libraries these days are much more than simply collections of documents. They provide a whole range of documents and services, Internet, CD-ROMs, videos, etc. The simple text-based interface has largely disappeared in conventional computing with the graphical user interface (GUI) based upon the desktop metaphor becoming almost ubiquitous.

The point-and-click interface used in the existing virtual libraries has superficial similarities to the Microsoft Windows interface used on most PCs across the world. However, it lacks the subtlety and depth of the desktop metaphor. In particular, users report difficulties in finding specific resources and in dealing with the wealth of information provided. Supporters of the current text-based point-and-click interface styles point to the vast growth of the Web as arguments for the status quo and point to the overheads associated with graphical interface types. It is interesting to note that almost 10 years ago (Gillies, 1991), the author was writing about a similar debate in end user computing applications with the defenders of command line interfaces making the same arguments against GUIs such as Windows.

There is a growing interest from librarians and practitioners in 'virtual libraries'. NHS initatives such as the National Electronic Library for Health and the NHS Information Zone are creating a much broader user base. Journals such as *Health Libraries Review* are publishing material on this subject (Gillies, 1999b). Others are questioning the role and purpose of virtual libraries in the health context (Guedon, 1999). These debates and the broader user base are challenging traditional assumptions about virtual libraries, their user models and the interface metaphors employed.

The rest of the paper describes a virtual health library developed at the Lancashire Postgraduate School of Medicine and Health (LPSMH) based upon a richer graphical metaphor and evaluates the end result in terms of traditional software quality criteria.

The LPSMH virtual health library

The LPSMH virtual health library (www.healthlibrary.org.uk/) has been developed principally for the support of students on the MSc Health Informatics programme, but is also intended for use by other health professionals and students within LPSMH.

The library is based around a graphical interface representing a room-based metaphor. The room metaphor has been used by other developers, notably Rank Xerox, who developed a commercial product based around such a metaphor a number of years ago.

On entering the library, you enter a front hall.

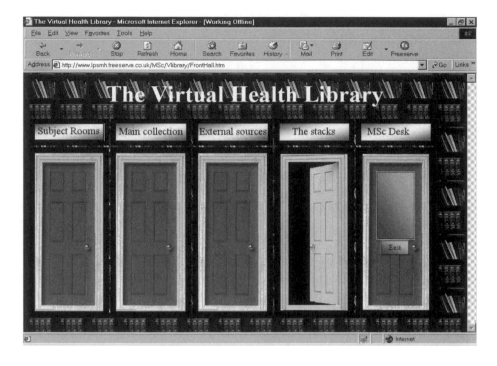

The use of books as a backdrop is intended to suggest a library ambience. The basic unit of the interface is the door. Three types of doors are used to signify movement around the library:

Panelled wooden doors   These are used to signify a metaphorical transition into another room within the library.

Semi glassed doors   These are used to signify a metaphorical transition into an area room outside of the library.

The open door   This is a special case, offering access to the metaphorical cellars where the stacks are stored. The cellars are part of the library but set apart (see below).

From here the user is guided through further doors to reach specific resources. For example, through the main collection door are three further rooms.

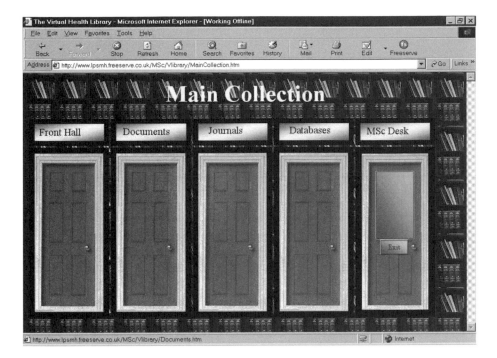

From here the user may access three 'rooms':

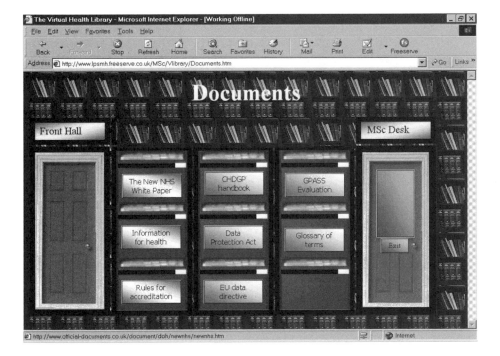

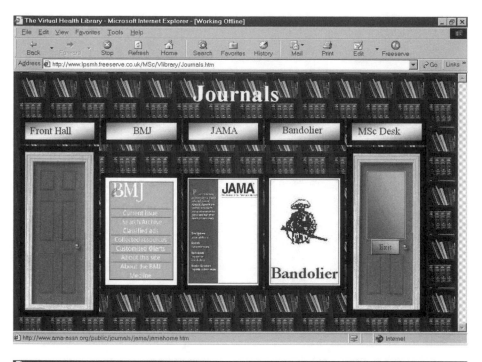

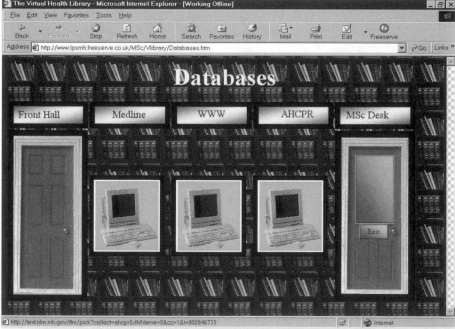

The metaphor is further underlined by the availability of a map. This gives you a map view of the layout which provides the twin benefits of reinforcing the spatial elements of the metaphor and providing rapid access to all parts of the library and MSc site through the use of hyperlinks direct to 'rooms':

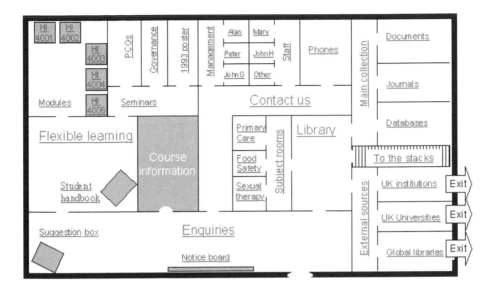

The second extended feature of the metaphor is the stacks. From interviews with potential users, the stacks is a fondly regarded feature of many academic libraries. The stacks is the archive collection of the library, often held in the cellar. It is a place where much information is held but where the user must search to find the information they require. In our virtual library, the stacks both reinforces the metaphor and serves to accommodate a much wider range of resources than are accommodated in the main library. A key concern to any educator in providing links to other sites must be the quality of the information, and the reliability of the links themselves. By establishing a stacks on a 'reader beware' basis, the educator is providing both an educational resource and an educational lesson.

Evaluation of the virtual library built upon the graphical metaphor

Traditional software evaluation has been based upon hierarchical models of quality criteria, such as those pioneered by McCall (1977, 1980), later adapted by Watts (1987), or Boehm (1981). In McCall's model, evaluation is based upon a set of criteria including usability, integrity, efficiency, correctness, reliability, maintainability, flexibility, testability, reusability, interoperability, and portability. The work by Watts (1987), demonstrated that these criteria could be clustered into groups. Work by the author (Gillies, 1992, 1997) has demonstrated that such criteria are in fact dependent upon a small set of measurable properties, such as structuredness, and that these properties are interrelated (Boehm, 1978; Gillies, 1997).

In considering evaluation criteria for these virtual libraries and noting the similarity in the debates between those over websites now and applications ten years ago, the author suggests a simplified version of the models cited above, recognising the closely related nature of the criteria in the models.

Therefore, we shall base our evaluation in terms of three characteristics:

- efficiency
- maintainability
- usability.

Traditionally, models such as those of Watts and McCall measured efficiency in terms of the size of lines of code designed to meet a desired goal. For years now, as hardware costs have dropped, efficiency has been sacrificed for usability and maintainability. However, in web terms, efficiency is again important as the download time for files makes performance a critical issue in everyday scenarios.

Efficiency of a website may be measured in terms of two key parameters. The first is the overall file size. Efficiency is inversely proportional to this. The second is the proportion of the site that uses material already downloaded. This is more tricky to assess, but the doors in the graphical metaphor, represent a potential for a graphical object that may be downloaded once, then reused.

Maintainability was traditionally seen as the inverse of the effort needed to make a change in the code, measured in terms of structure. This may be measured crudely in terms of the inverse of the number of lines of HTML. However, since download time is again crucial, it may also be logically seen as the size of the elements required to be changed to effect a change in the web page.

Usability has always been the hardest to measure, and requires user trials to make definitive judgements, combining tests of user reaction to the interface with tests of their ability to use it without error. At the design stage of a web page, however, there are a number of key issues, which can be considered including:

- consistency of metaphor and mental model
- depth of metaphor and mental model
- speed of access to all elements of the site.

A crucial aspect of the author's earlier work with application quality was the recognition of non-commutative relationships between the quality criteria (Gillies, 1992). It was shown that the criteria were often in conflict. Thus, increasing the structuredness of the code would increase maintainability, but reduce efficiency. The use of GUIs compared to command-line interfaces increased usability at the expense of efficiency. The relationships for our three key criteria in terms of applications were as follows (*see* Table 7.1; Gillies, 1992):

Table 7.1 Relationships between quality criteria for applications

Maintainability	Efficiency	Maintainability	Usability
Efficiency		−	−
Maintainability	−		−
Usability	−	0	

Source: Gillies, 1992.

The table expresses relationships in the manner first devised by Boehm (1981). A (+) indicates that if quality in terms of criteria A is improved, then quality in terms of criteria B is likely to be improved.

However, for web pages we have a different picture. Since the two key factors in efficiency, file compactness and percentage available for reuse, are both positively influenced by structure, then maintainability and efficiency are likely to be reinforcing rather than conflicting (*see* Table 7.2).

Table 7.2 Relationships between quality criteria for web pages

	Efficiency	Maintainability	Usability
Efficiency		+	−
Maintainability	+		−
Usability	−	0	

To test the evaluation and to consider the differences between different metaphors, we shall use the above criteria to evaluate the relative performance of three versions of the virtual library.

Version 1 is a 'point-and-click' version of the library, developed solely for comparison.

Version 2 uses the full graphical metaphor as implemented at the time of writing (June 1999), which was shown on p. 64.

Version 3 is an earlier graphical version, developed using Microsoft Powerpoint 97.

The three versions of the front hall page are shown below. Whilst there are some version differences between versions 2 and 3, these are normalised in the analysis. The parameters used to generate version 3 in terms of graphical format (.jpg) and resolution (640 × 480 for main image) are set to match those of version 2.

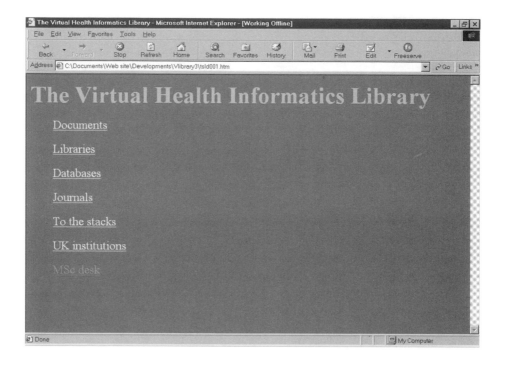

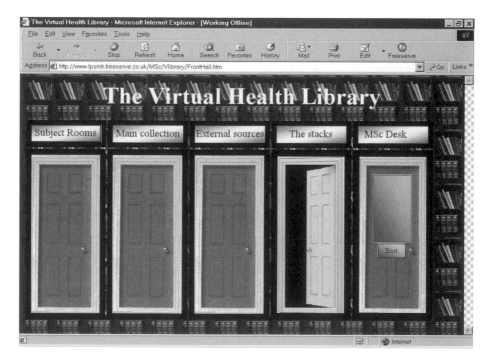

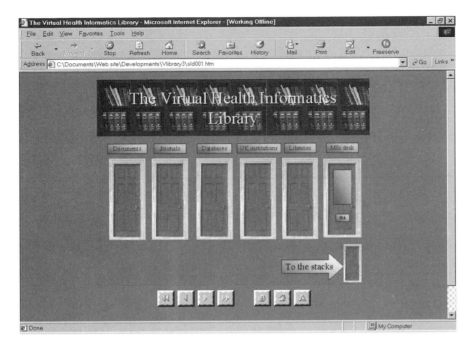

Using the criteria noted above, Table 7.3 indicates relative performance, in terms of each of the efficiency and maintainability criteria defined above, of key pages within the virtual library for the three versions detailed. In the charts below performance is normalised against the performance of the worst case on each occasion.

Table 7.3   Analysis of the websites in terms of the criteria specified

| | Efficiency | | | | | | Maintainability | | | | | |
| | File size | | | Reuse | | | Lines of HTML | | | Size of elements required | | |
Version	1	2	3	1	2	3	1	2	3	1	2	3
Front page	1	90	280	0	45	0	25	28	44	1	14	280
Documents	1	92	229	0	77	0	25	48	44	1	14	229
Journals	1	62	241	0	33	0	25	28	44	1	14	241
Databases	1	75	205	0	32	0	24	28	42	1	14	205
UK institutions	1	94	263	0	73	0	25	28	44	1	14	263
Global libraries	1	90	252	0	73	0	25	27	44	1	14	252

Raw analysis in terms of file sizes only (*see* Figure 7.1) shows that although the optimised graphical version improves over the automatically generated version, it remains markedly less efficient than the text version. However, the optimisation is better reflected if we take account of the ability of web browsers to cache elements locally. The relative performance of the optimised version then improves dramatically (*see* Figure 7.2).

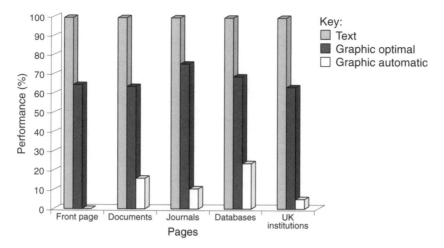

Figure 7.1 Efficiency of virtual library site.

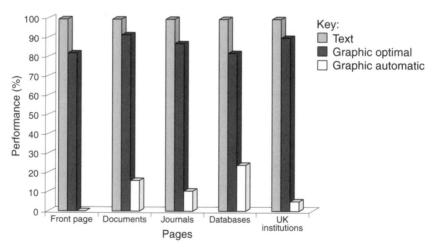

Figure 7.2 Efficiency of virtual library site including reuse.

Apart from the first load of the very first page, this measure is a better measure of practical efficiency. It indicates practical estimated load times of .03 second, one second, and nine seconds for typical pages in the three versions respectively.

In terms of maintainability, raw measures in terms of lines of code give little indication of real issues. However, it should be noted that the documents page of the optimised graphical version is significantly larger than the other files. However, more significant is the size of the element required to make a change, both in terms of finding an error and uploading the new version. Maintainability measured in this way is shown in Figure 7.3.

As noted, it is harder to measure usability at the design stage. Formal usability trials are planned for the future. However, the site has been made available to a

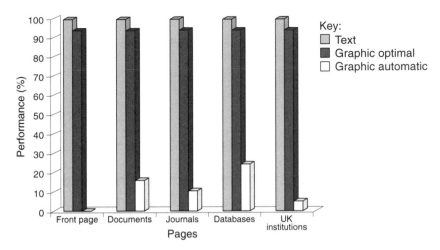

Figure 7.3 Maintainability in terms of time to reload changes.

range of potential users with limited IT expertise, including counsellors, food safety managers and a clinical consultant. Comments from users, such as 'I can relate to this', 'I would actually use this', 'this is excellent – I can find my way around', suggest the richness of the metaphor is appreciated by users.

Discussion

The virtual library community has grown up within the community of web enthusiasts. It has therefore adopted the limited document text-based metaphor for its own use. The use of point-and-click interfaces has allowed this to be portrayed to the wider community as an extension of the GUIs used on nearly all desktops. However, the poverty of the metaphor has produced significant problems amongst some users.

This study has sought to demonstrate how a richer metaphor can be employed with major advantages to novice users without unreasonable compromises in terms of performance. It has shown that the optimisation of implementation can produce efficiency and maintainability results much closer to those of text-based websites than to those generated automatically with little optimisation.

The parallels with debates in software development from ten years ago are instructive. At the point where the efficiency issues became insignificant, maintainability and usability of such systems came to the fore. This led to the current vogue for GUIs, structured programming and rapid application development, often using visual programming environments. It may be argued, therefore, that where richer graphical metaphors can be implemented efficiently, then they will become the norm even for the more utilitarian websites such as virtual health libraries.

In terms of quality criteria, the most significant difference between software quality criteria then and website quality now is that in optimising websites for efficiency, it is likely that maintainability will also be enhanced, because of the pivotal role that download times play in the use of websites. This is in contrast to conventional software experience where efficiency has often been achieved at the expense of maintainability.

Conclusions

The paper started by noting the metaphorical poverty of many virtual health libraries on the Web. The study has shown how a library based upon a richer metaphor can be developed and implemented in an efficient manner.

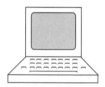

On-line resource
If you visit the library today, you will find it has developed dramatically, but retains the principles on which it was founded. The library is accessible in the Chapter 7 section of the website accompanying this book.

On-line resources

Evaluating on-line resources requires us to evaluate the site and its content. We shall visit a range of websites and evaluate them using a series of criteria.

Site criteria

- Visual appeal: Does it look attractive?
- Ease of navigation: Is there a logical path through the site?
- Efficiency: Do the pages load quickly?
- Layout: Is there a simple layout without clutter?
- Consistent: Is the interface consistent in its use of icons, fonts and metaphor?
- Reliability: Does it work without error, and without 'dead' links?

Content criteria

- Accuracy: Does it appear to provide accurate information?
- Honesty: Does it warn of possible biases?
- Evidential basis: Does it provide evidence for its arguments, or distinguish between peer-reviewed information and non peer-reviewed information?

- Usefulness: Is the content useful?
- Feedback: Is there an opportunity to contact the author to report errors or make comments?

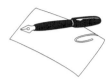

Practical activities

Visit each site listed below. You may like to use the table below to help you with your evaluation, rating each site according to the following scale:

1   very poor
2   poor
3   adequate
4   good
5   very good.

Make a note as you go through of useful resources found.

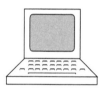

On-line resources
All of the sites to be evaluated are available through the Chapter 7 section of the website accompanying this book. The grids are also available in printable form.

Site criteria

Site	Visual appeal	Ease of navigation	Efficiency	Layout	Consistency	Reliability
Virtual library						
NHS Direct						
NLM						
Health Canada						
Department of Health						
NHSIA						
NICE						
BMJ						
JAMA						
Bandolier						

Content criteria

Site	Accuracy	Honesty	Evidential basis	Usefulness	Feedback
Virtual library					
NHS Direct					
NLM					
Health Canada					
Department of Health					
NHSIA					
NICE					
BMJ					
JAMA					
Bandolier					

Useful resources

Site	Useful resources
Virtual library	
NHS Direct	
NLM	
Health Canada	
Department of Health	
NHSIA	
NICE	
BMJ	
JAMA	
Bandolier	

Key points

By the end of this section, you should be able to:

1 Have an appreciation of the range of on-line sources available on the Web.
2 Be able to evaluate on-line sources.
3 Be able to track down useful information using the World Wide Web.

8

Information strategy for PCOs: the GPIMM model

Introduction

In this chapter we shall consider information strategy planning for practices and the PCO. To start, visit the on-line seminar on the information needs of PCOs, which includes a description of GPIMM ca 1997, then look at a more recent presentation made to the National Association of Primary Care (NAPC) in 2001.

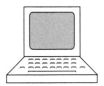

On-line resource
These presentations are available through the Chapter 8 section of the website accompanying this book.

Using GPIMM for PCO information strategy planning

The starting point for implementing an information strategy across the PCO is to carry out an audit of the general practices within your group. However, you are not starting from scratch. The health authority should already hold the basic practice information. This will include the following information about the practice itself:

- name and number of practice
- address(es) of surgery
- telephone and fax numbers
- practice number (where applicable).

It will include the following information about the partners and staff:

- name
- professional identification (ID) numbers
- role details
- contractual relationships with dates.

It will include the following information about related organisations:

- name and identification (ID) number
- address
- telephone and fax numbers
- contact details of key personnel.

And hopefully also the following about the practice information system:

- supplier
- version
- coding system and version.

The first step in making progress is to establish how developed the practices are in terms of their use of information. We have developed a model for such a purpose, and we will use it to establish development plans for every practice in order to enable them to contribute to the PCO information system.

The model is known as the GPIMM, the General Practice Information Maturity Model. We shall use a simplified version of the model to illustrate how it works.

The model defines where a practice is in terms of a maturity level. You may like to think of this as a step on a staircase leading to the level required for the practice to play a full part in the PCO information system.

This is why you will find a staircase as the logo of the model (*see* Figure 8.1). The model is based around five primary maturity levels, with an additional zero level for non-computerised practices. The maturity levels are summarised in Table 8.1.

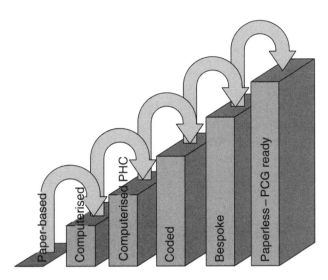

Figure 8.1 Five attainable steps from paper-based to paperless practice.

Table 8.1 Levels of the GPIMM

Level	Designation	Summary description
0	Paper-based	The practice has no computer system
1	Computerised	The practice has a computer system. It is used only by the practice staff
2	Computerised PHC team	The practice has a computer system. It is used by the practice staff and the PHC team, including the doctors
3	Coded	The system makes limited use of Read codes
4	Bespoke	The system is tailored to the needs of the practice through agreed coding policies and the use of clinical protocols
5	Paperless	The practice is completely paperless, except where paper records are a legal requirement

The model can help with two key tasks: identifying where practices are, and what they need to do to make progress. In this chapter we shall consider how to use the GPIMM to audit where practices are.

The audit is based around a relatively simple questionnaire. This is possible because the model has at its heart a logical model of practice information development. Practices that show different levels of maturity in different areas should consider whether those developments have occurred in a logical fashion.

The presence of 'outliers', i.e. higher or lower maturity levels in one area may be indicative of wasted efforts.

The questionnaire considers five areas to assess maturity.

Computerisation: This is simply a filter to identify those practices that remain paper based.

Personnel usage: This section looks at the impact of the system upon the practice. Systems used only by practice staff are severely limited in their usefulness.

Coding: This section is crucial. It considers not just the extent of coding, but the quality of coding through the extent of policies and consultation underpinning coding practice.

System usage: This section is concerned with the impact that the system has upon the working methods of the practice. It measures the extent to which the system works for the practice and not the other way around.

Electronic patient records (EPR):   This section is concerned with the implementation of the EPR. It considers how far the EPR is realised both inside and outside the practice.

A simplified version of the questionnaire is included below.

GPIMM maturity level questionnaire

Computerisation
Has the practice got a computerised patient record system installed?

Yes   No

If No, simply return the questionnaire now.

Personnel usage
Is the system in use within the practice?

Yes   No

Is the system used by doctors and other members of the primary healthcare team during consultations?

Yes   No

Coding
Is any information Read coded by users of the system?

Yes   No

Has the whole practice adopted standard Read codes for key clinical areas?

Yes   No

Are the codes entered subject to a validation procedure?

Yes   No

Has the practice liaised with other stakeholders such as other practices within commissioning groups, or the health authority over standard Read codes?

Yes   No

Has the practice adopted a policy of 100% coding on patient records?

Yes   No

System usage
Is the system used to proactively manage repeat prescribing?

Yes   No

Is the system used to proactively manage acute prescribing?

Yes   No

Is the system used to proactively manage health promotion?

Yes   No

Is the system used to implement clinical protocols?

Yes   No

Is the system used to carry out real time audits?

Yes   No

Electronic patient records
Is the system electronically linked to the PCO for transferring information on items of service?

Yes   No

Is the system fully linked to NHSnet?

Yes   No

Are paper records only used when legally required?

Yes   No

The easiest way to assess a GPIMM maturity level is to use one of the software tools available to implement the model.

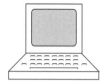

On-line resource
The Chapter 8 section of the website accompanying this book has a demonstration tool, GPIMM-CAPA (General Practice Information Maturity Model-Computer Aided Practice Assessment tool). This software runs under Windows 95 on any PC. The GPIMM-CAPA provides an electronic version of the questionnaire together with an assessment of the current maturity level and further information to be used for practice development.

The commercial version of the software, based upon the latest version of GPIMM, is provided as an Access database for PCOs combined with a training needs analysis tool.

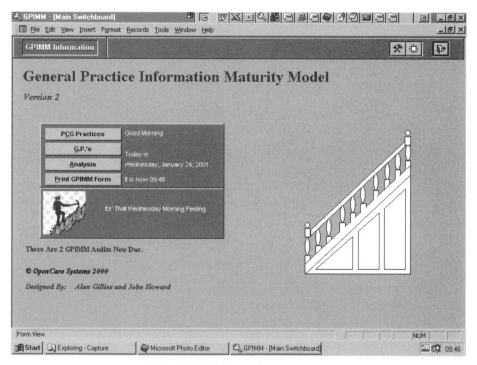

The GPIMM opening screen.

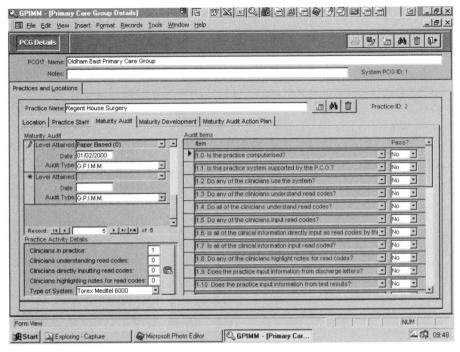

The GPIMM audit.

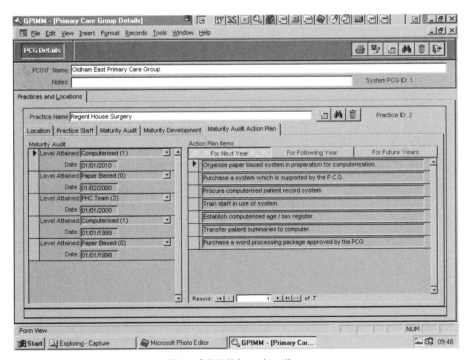

The GPIMM action list.

Using the GPIMM it is possible to build a profile of the practice or target PCO audience. A simple graph will show at a glance the scale of the problem.

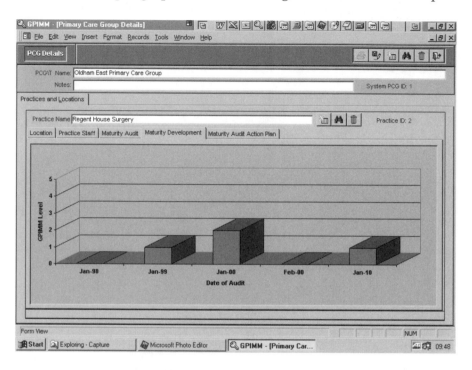

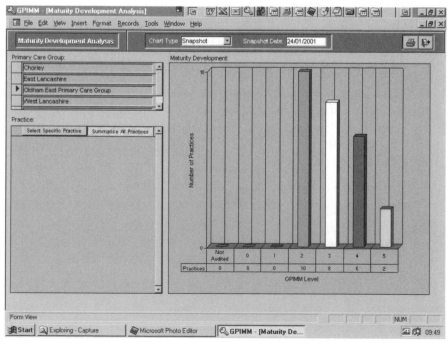

Audits of local practices have typically shown the majority of practices at Levels 2 and 3 leaving a lot of work to be done.

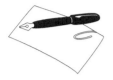

Practical activities

Using the GPIMM-CAPA tool carry out a GPIMM audit of your practice, what level do you achieve?

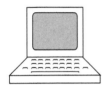

On-line resource
The Chapter 8 section of the website accompanying this book has links to the GPIMM website for the latest information. It also provides access to 'making it happen' in the IT section of www.primarycareonline.co.uk, Module 8 of which has a GPIMM case study. (Also found in Gillies, 1999a.)

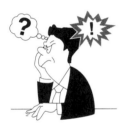

Questions to think about

Before we consider using GPIMM for practice development, think about the following:

GPIMM-CAPA will indicate what tasks are priorities for practice information development. Before moving on, draw up your own list to see if you agree.

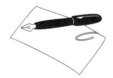

Practical activities

Practice X is a practice of 10 000 patients with five doctors. The practice prides itself on being innovative, and was a first wave fundholding practice. It is based in a suburban area, with new premises developed since the practice became fundholding. The practice is interested in developing health promotion activities and is currently seeking to implement an ischaemic heart disease programme.

They are currently using an IPS computer system. The system is based around the old text-based Medical System with additional modules for items of service. The practice is linked to the health authority for items of service information.

The system is currently used within consultations by the doctors. Repeat and acute prescriptions are handled by the computer system. However, none of the information is currently coded. The usage of the system is as a basic recording device with little proactive usage.

Use the GPIMM-CAPA to see what level of maturity is currently achieved. Draw up an action plan for this practice to reach the required level for participation in the PCO. Enter the action plan in the table below.

Year	GPIMM level	Tasks to be carried out

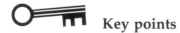 **Key points**

By the end of this section, you should be able to:

1   Understand the principles underpinning the GPIMM model.
2   Audit a practice using the GPIMM-CAPA tool.
3   Draw up practice improvement plans using GPIMM-CAPA.

9

Quality assurance

Introduction

The purpose of this chapter is to establish the context of quality assurance in healthcare, of which clinical governance is the current manifestation. The basis of a framework for assessing current performance will be established and the nature of patient care, in terms of defining its quality, will be explored. The chapter starts with the general problem of defining quality and then considers the specific area of healthcare and its particular characteristics.

The concept of 'views' of quality is introduced through the specific example of the care of expectant mothers, considering the principal stakeholders and their views. The general model of Garvin is then considered and its appropriateness for healthcare reviewed. This is followed by a model derived from Garvin's original, but tailored for healthcare. The chapter concludes with a consideration of the conflicts and constraints upon quality using this latter model as a basis.

What is quality?

Some of the simplest questions are the most difficult to answer. 'What is quality?' ranks with the most difficult of them. In domains such as engineering, quality may be linked to tangible physical properties. However, in many other areas (e.g. patient care in medicine) quality is intangible. As Kitchenham (1989) said in a different context, quality in such cases is 'hard to define, impossible to measure, easy to recognise'.

Quality is most easily recognised in its absence, and many public perceptions of healthcare are based upon measuring the absence of quality, for example, waiting times, waiting list sizes, even illness itself are all measurements of the absence of quality.

Traditionally, quality has been seen as 'the degree of excellence' (OED, 1990). This is an attractive definition but is insufficient for our purposes. The nature of 'excellence' must be considered in more detail to make the definition more effective. However, there is a more serious problem with this definition. Within a public health service context, it is necessary to consider the constraints upon excellence. Obviously, the primary constraint is budget, but others may exist, for example, shortage of specialist skills in clinical specialties or nursing.

An alternative definition of quality is provided by the International Standards Organization (ISO):

'The totality of features and characteristics of a product or service that bear on its ability to satisfy specified or implied needs' (ISO, 1994).

The standard definition associates quality with the ability of the product or service to fulfil its function. It recognises that this is achieved through the features and characteristics of the product. Quality is associated both with having the required range of attributes and achieving satisfactory performance within each attribute. It is important to recognise some of the primary characteristics of quality:

Quality is not absolute. It means different things in different situations. In the case of cars, a Mini and a Rolls-Royce both represent quality in different ways. Quality cannot be measured upon a quantifiable scale in the same way as physical properties such as temperature or length.

Quality is multidimensional. It has many contributing factors. It is not easily summarised in a simple, quantitative way. Some aspects of quality can be measured objectively, e.g. time spent waiting to see a doctor; some may not, e.g. quality of a doctor's manner during a consultation. The most easily measured criteria are not necessarily the most important. People are irrational beings, and the acceptability of their treatment may depend upon criteria which are very hard to define.

Quality is subject to constraints. Assessment of quality in most cases cannot be separated from cost. However, cost may be wider than simple financial cost; it refers to any critical resources such as people, tools and time. Some resources will be more constrained than others and where there is a high demand for a resource that is heavily constrained, the availability of that resource will become critical to overall quality.

Quality is about acceptable compromises. Where quality is constrained and compromises are required, some quality criteria may be sacrificed more acceptably than others, e.g. comfort may be sacrificed before productivity. Those criteria that can least afford to be sacrificed may be regarded as critical attributes. They are often a small subset of the overall set of quality criteria.

Quality criteria are not independent. The quality criteria are not independent, but interact with each other causing conflicts. For example, the greater the number of patients assigned to a clinic, the longer the waiting time during the clinic, but the shorter the waiting time to get an appointment. In this case, a conflict exists between the two desirable attributes.

Acceptable quality changes over time. Progress in clinical practice and improvements in care mean that levels of performance deemed to be satisfactory are constantly being raised. This is an increase in both actual capability and in public expectation.

Definitions from within medicine

The problem of defining quality in medical terms is the complexity of the issue. Any domain where we are dealing with people rather than artefacts is infinitely more complex. Many authors say that looking at improving healthcare through a quality assurance model derived from the manufacturing industry is inappropriate:

'*human well-being and the healthcare industry which deals with it are infinitely more complex than production lines*' (Crombie *et al.*, 1993).

As far as it goes, this statement is fine, but quality assurance is now applied in many different organisational and service contexts which face many of the same issues as healthcare, e.g. education.

The difficulty is in not oversimplifying the issues. This is particularly true when we try to express the quality of healthcare in terms of simple quantitative measures.

For example, one traditional measure of healthcare is morbidity data. Many such measures tend to emphasise issues of quantity rather than quality. Clinicians who tend to evaluate themselves in terms of the quality of patients' lives rather than the quantity of it are uncomfortable with this.

In practice, most writers in the clinical domain choose not to define quality at all, unless dealing with a very specific and tightly defined area. For example, the definition of clinical audit provided by the Department of Health states:

'*the systematic, critical analysis of the quality of medical care, including the procedures used for diagnosis and treatment, the use of resources and the resulting outcome and quality of life for the patient*' (DoH, 1990).

This definition contains the phrases 'quality of medical care' and 'quality of life' but nowhere defines what is meant by these terms. There is a broad consensus about general characteristics associated with these terms but at a detailed level, different clinicians and other interested parties, not least patients, are likely to disagree. Therefore, rather than attempt a reductionist definition different views of the quality of patient care in a specific context will be considered. In the next section, we shall consider the situation relating to the care of mothers, from the antenatal to postnatal period.

Views of quality

It is important to recognise that quality is a multidimensional construct. Therefore, it is perhaps inevitable that it has been classified according to a number of 'views' or perspectives. This is represented by a visual analogy (*see* Figure 9.1).

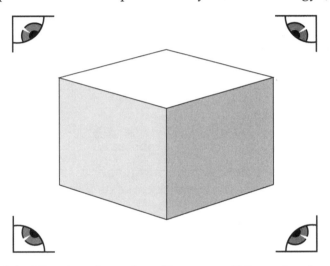

Figure 9.1   Visual analogy of quality as a multidimensional construct.

These views are often diverse and may conflict with each other. Each view comes from a particular context, and any single view may give only a partial picture. The views identified tend to be stereotypical. For example, a distinction is commonly made within the Health Service context between the clinicians or professionals and the managers or administrators. The views are generally presented in adversarial pairs, such as professionals versus administrators. Such comparisons are usually loaded by the terminology used.

Obviously, there are more than two people involved in any healthcare procedure. The care of postnatal patients is particularly interesting for a number of reasons:

- it involves an unusually large number of people in different roles dealing with the patient
- the patient is generally not ill.

Each of the following roles and their view of quality will be considered:

• the mother
• the hospital midwife
• the doctor
• the community midwife
• the baby
• the unit manager
• the mother's partner.

The mother

The mother's view of the quality of her experience will depend on two factors: a successful outcome and a positive experience before, during and after the birth. The duality of this view is emphasised by the fact that most mothers are not ill. Obviously at some points, these views are reinforcing. A simple and successful birth will encourage a positive view of the whole experience. However, some procedures which may be deemed clinically desirable to maximise the probability of a successful outcome may be highly invasive and disturbing for the mother.

Increasingly, the separation between these aspects is being questioned as it is recognised that clinical outcomes are influenced by a patient's general state of well-being. This increases the need to take account of what have been traditionally considered as non-clinical aspects of care.

The hospital midwife

The hospital midwife is, in fact, responsible for most births. The multidisciplinary approach which is recognised in many clinical specialties as desirable has been reality in delivering babies for a long time. The hospital midwife's prime responsibility is for a successful outcome for mother and baby. Their view of quality is complicated by their dual responsibility to both mother and baby. Increasingly, they are also being influenced by a need to demonstrate that all eventualities were considered in the light of possible litigation in the event of problems. This theme is discussed later.

The doctor

Doctors are generally only involved significantly in births that have clinical complications. One doctor remarked that this made her an awful expectant mother as she had only ever witnessed difficult births. This, coupled with the fact that the doctor carries ultimate responsibility for any clinical problems will tend to emphasise a view of quality based upon clinical outcomes.

The community midwife

The community midwife may be involved at the birth in the event of a home delivery, but is more likely to be responsible for the daily postnatal care of mother and baby. They tend to avoid the worst clinical complications, and therefore can afford to pay more attention to the patients' comfort. Since they are generally involved postnatally, they will also deal overtly with mother and baby.

The baby

The baby, although unable to express a view, is the focus of at least half the care provided. Once again, there are clinical and experiential aspects of the quality of care received. However, the clinical aspects often dominate as the baby is not able to vocalise objections to treatments that may be thought clinically desirable, but are unpleasant for the baby.

The unit manager

The manager of the unit has the job of ensuring the quality of patient care delivered. Crucially, they have to weigh the needs of all patients rather than individuals. They have to weigh decisions against available resources and this leads to having to evaluate the quality of care against the quantity.

The mother's partner

Partners of mothers generally have a direct and indirect interest in the process, although the roles may be distinct. As the father of the child, they have a direct interest in the successful birth of their offspring. As the mother's partner they have an interest in both the mother's health and happiness. Decisions to exclude partners from parts of the process, particularly at the antenatal stage, on the grounds of clinical expediency can lead to dissatisfaction and resentment.

Modelling views of quality

Within the general management context, Garvin (1984) has suggested a model in terms of five different views of quality (*see* Figure 9.2).

The meaning of Garvin's views are summarised in Table 9.1.

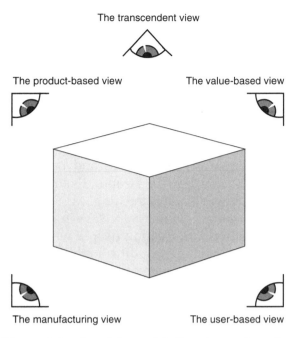

The transcendent view

The product-based view   The value-based view

The manufacturing view   The user-based view

Figure 9.2 Garvin's model: five views of quality.

Table 9.1 Summary of Garvin's views of quality	
View	*Meaning*
Transcendent	Absolute excellence
Product-based	Higher quality means higher cost
User-based	Fitness for purpose
Manufacturing	Conformance to specification
Value-based	Quality at a specific price

These views are now considered in more detail within the context of healthcare.

The transcendent view

This view relates quality to innate excellence. Another word for this might be 'elegance'. This is the classical definition of quality, in tune with the Oxford English Dictionary. It is impossible to quantify and is difficult to apply in a meaningful sense to healthcare. An attempt to build in a high degree of innate excellence in healthcare is likely to be constrained by resources. Seeking to build healthcare along these lines is inevitably expensive, and thus resource constraints will tend to emphasise the value-based view, described opposite, rather than the transcendent view.

The product-based view

This view is the economist's view: the higher the quality, the higher the cost. The basis for this view is that it costs money to provide a higher quality. This is a commonly held view about healthcare. Better care and quicker access to services are commonly linked to more doctors, nurses and hospital beds. However, in certain areas, better practice may also be cheaper. Examples of this may be found in screening programmes where health screening, e.g. for blood pressure, cervical cancer and child immunisation, can actually save money in the long-term by keeping people healthy rather than treating people when they become ill.

Also, the growing practice of clinical audit is highlighting areas where practice can be improved without necessarily increasing costs. This is the classic 'quality is free' argument translated from manufacturing to healthcare, proposed by, for example, Crosby (1986). Crosby argues that by changing practice and reducing wastage, savings can be achieved in manufacturing which outweigh the costs of setting up the new procedures. However, unfortunately, this is by no means universal. Many improved practices will involve new technology requiring investment. Once wastage is removed, improvements in waiting lists can only be achieved by more resources.

Many of the screening programmes which are cost effective in the long-term are expensive in the short-term. For example, the growth in screening programmes in the UK has driven up computerisation rates amongst family doctors from around 25% to 90%. This represents a major investment where cost must be set against the savings as illness is reduced. Further, if screening programmes are justified on cost grounds alone, then programmes advantageous to health, but less advantageous on cost grounds, may be marginalised, e.g. breast cancer screening. From a health perspective, it is still better to prevent illness rather than treat it, but this case conforms to Garvin's product-based view, i.e. higher quality of care costs more.

The user-based view

This view, first championed by Juran in the 1940s, is traditionally expressed as 'fitness for purpose' (Juran, 1979). It is sometimes represented as patient satisfaction. However, this can be a simplification.

Fitness for purpose implies that the service provided meets the needs of patients, considering certain aspects of performance such as waiting times, access to services and patient satisfaction. However, overall fitness for purpose is compromised if waiting times are reduced by emphasising the treatment of conditions that are quick, easy and cheap at the expense of more seriously ill patients.

It is also compromised if waiting times are reduced at the expense of reducing the effectiveness of treatment provided leading to an increase in readmissions. Many measures currently applied to the UK NHS which purport to measure NHS fitness for purpose, e.g. waiting times, waiting list sizes, number of patients treated, actually measure the quantity of healthcare provided rather than the quality.

The manufacturing view

The manufacturer's view measures quality in terms of conformance to requirements. A simple example might be the dimensions of a component. The specification will state both the required dimension and the tolerance that will be acceptable.

The manufacturing view emerges in healthcare in a number of ways. The first is the introduction of protocols and standards for specific clinical procedures. These may be regarded as a specification for a clinical procedure. In the UK, one of the stated outcomes of the clinical audit process is the introduction of standards to disseminate 'best practice'.

However, the setting of such standards is by no mean universal; a report on audit practice in the Oxfordshire Health Authority revealed that only 46% of audits were claimed to result in the setting of standards (Anglia & Oxford RHA and NHSE, 1994). Evaluation of 75 published audits indicated a 41% uptake. As published audits, these may be expected to show a higher uptake than the whole, suggesting that the real figure may be lower.

In practice, it is rarely possible to provide guidelines which embody 'best practice'. Guidelines will prevent bad practice and can lead to uniform improvements where existing practice is flawed. However, best practice generally requires skills and judgement rather than following deterministic procedures. The biggest threat to this lies in the increasing threat of malpractice suits. This encourages doctors to view quality in terms of meeting a specification. If the specification is met, the doctor has fulfilled his obligation, even if the patients' aspirations are not met. Thus the result of guidelines can be problem avoidance rather than promotion of excellence.

The value-based view

In a business context, this is the ability to provide what the customer requires at a price that they can afford. In a public health service, the customer is ultimately the taxpaying public represented by the Government. A value-based view of quality assesses the cost-effectiveness of a service or treatment.

The value-based view is the antithesis of the transcendent view, because it links quality to cost. Within the management of quality in the NHS context, this is often the crucial view. It is also what tends to give NHS management a bad name in the eyes of the public, as it recognises that quality is ultimately resource-limited. Although there are cases where better healthcare costs less not more, as described above, in general this is not the case.

Garvin's model is not necessarily appropriate for healthcare. For example, the manufacturing view which is dominant in many areas of traditional quality management is of limited use. The author therefore proposes an alternative view-based model of quality for healthcare (*see* Figure 9.3).

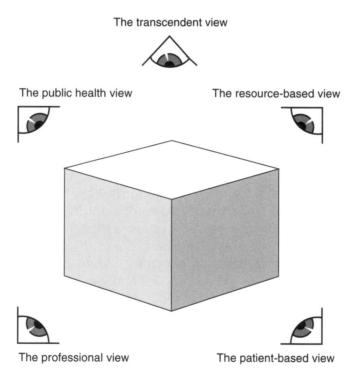

Figure 9.3   A view-based model of the quality of patient care.

The transcendent view

This view is the same as Garvin's. It is included because it is such a deeply ingrained view of quality. It is of little help in analysing the problem of improving the quality of patient care. However, it is important to recognise its crucial place in many people's understanding of the nature of quality.

The public health view

This view is based upon the belief that the quality of patient care is demonstrated by the health of the nation. It is the view at the heart of the UK Government's strategy documents, *Health of the Nation* (DoH, 1992a) and *Our Healthier Nation* (DoH, 1998c), which set targets for key areas.

A key element of this view is that quality of care is reflected in maintaining and restoring health rather than through treating illness. This view may be seen as a strategic view of the quality of patient care.

The resource-based view

The resource-based view says that the quality of patient care is the maximum care that can be obtained for the resources allocated by the country to public healthcare. It is concerned with the effectiveness of patient care, reduction of waste and promotion of best practice measured in terms of value for money. This may be thought of as the management view, at both an operational and strategic level.

The professional view

This view emphasises clinical outcomes and clinical expertise. It sets a successful clinical outcome as the primary measure of success. Traditionally, it has emphasised the central role of the doctor, but it is now beginning to promote a team-based approach. However, some doctors may use a narrow form of this view to resist change in this direction. It is a view associated with doctors and other clinical professionals.

The patient-based view

The patient-based view says that the patients' overall well-being and satisfaction is crucial. It tends to an individualistic view rather than a collective vision, as the needs of each patient may be different and conflict, under the resource-based view, with the needs of other patients. In certain cases it may also conflict with the professional view. However, many professionals placing their patients needs as their prime objective, will subscribe to this view, although expressing it in a different way from the patients they seek to serve.

These views are necessarily stereotypical, as any model must represent a subset of reality. They are intended to be less stereotypical than a reductionist definition and more appropriate to healthcare than Garvin's general model. We shall return to them in later chapters.

Conflicts and constraints

There is an extra degree of complexity inherent in this model which arises from the relationships which exist between each view of quality. It is suggested that each of the views except the transcendent view is in dynamic equilibrium with the others. The equilibrium is dynamic because many improvements as perceived from one point of view may degrade quality when perceived from another point of view. Each of the other four contributes to the transcendent view.

The dynamic equilibrium may be thought of in terms of a variety of conflicts between different views (*see* Figure 9.4).

The most commonly considered conflict is between cost and quality, or in terms of our views between the resource-based view and the public health view. Any improvements which can impact positively on more than one view without negatively impacting elsewhere are particularly attractive. Some of the screening programmes mentioned earlier are in this category.

However, there are other conflicts at work between the different views. There is a significant and growing conflict between patient- and professional-based views. A better informed public arising from a more patient-centred approach argues more strongly for their rights, and attacks the traditionally unquestioned expertise of the professionals.

Part of this is a growing awareness of the right of patients to make charges of negligence in cases where things go wrong. This has a number of consequences, but one is that doctors may take courses of action in order to protect themselves against malpractice suits rather than for patient-centred reasons. This will then tend to reduce the quality in terms of the patient-based approach. This is more evident in the USA, where litigation is much more common than in the UK.

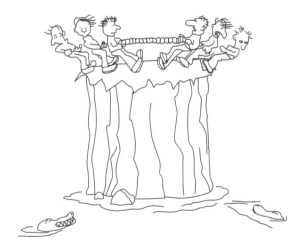

Figure 9.4 Conflict between different views.

The behaviour of American obstetricians is an example of this approach. In the face of the increasing incidence of malpractice suits over birth canal deliveries they have opted for an increased number of Caesarean section deliveries. In spite of the increased risk to patients, this was less likely to lead to a law suit. At its peak, this trend led to approximately 50% of babies being delivered by Caesarean section. However, this was followed by a series of law suits which alleged unnecessary Caesarean operations, which in turn reduced the number of operations. This slightly bizarre example illustrates the dynamic equilibrium which exists between different views of quality.

In an ideal world, all views would be satisfied, leading to the transcendent view of quality. However, in the real world, all of the others exist in different degrees of tension with each other. This is what makes a discussion of the quality of patient care so difficult and makes a multidimensional treatment essential.

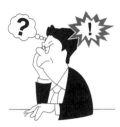

Questions to think about

1   How far are the views discussed above represented within clinical governance policy?
2   In what circumstances is the highest quality of care provided by over-ruling the wishes of the patients?

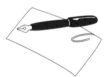

Practical activities

Investigate the clinical governance plans for your organisation. Consider how they reflect the views of quality that we have discussed here.

   Key points

By the end of this section, you should be able to:

1   Understand that quality is a relative construct, dependent upon the viewpoint of the observer.
2   Understand that different views of quality may conflict.
3   Understand how interventions to improve quality may have the opposite effect.

10

Introduction to clinical governance

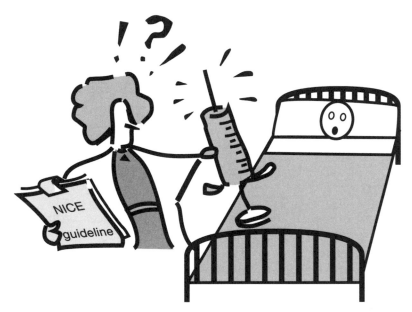

'This is going to hurt me more than it will hurt you.'

Introduction

This chapter is designed to introduce clinical governance.

Clinical governance

Before reading this chapter, you will need to read the following:

Department of Health (1997) *The New NHS White Paper*.
Department of Health (1998) *A First Class Service*.

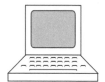

On-line resource
The Chapter 10 section of the website accompanying this book has links to these two key documents.

Also read the following briefing paper.

The evolution of healthcare quality assurance within the NHS: from clinical audit to clinical governance

Introduction

The development of systematic quality assurance practices within the UK NHS may be viewed in terms of three distinct phases. Prior to 1990, quality assurance was essentially regarded as part of the professionalism of individual clinicians.

In 1990, for the first time, clinical audit was made a normal part of every clinician's professional duties (DoH, 1989a). However, it remained ad hoc and no attempt to introduce systematic quality assurance was made. In particular, professional practice was not made subject to any external review.

In 1997, following the election of a new Government, a new wave of NHS reforms was introduced (DoH, 1997). These included the introduction of clinical governance, a systematic process of quality assurance. Whilst this was being discussed, a major scandal broke in Bristol, which has forced the external scrutiny of professional practice to be introduced (Dyer, 1998; Smith, 1998).

In this paper, we shall present a critical analysis of the evolution of quality assurance through these distinct phases, and use the analysis to develop a strategic framework for clinical governance.

The evolution of healthcare quality assurance in the UK up to 1990

Clinicians have always had professional interest in the quality of their work. However, early studies were isolated research studies such as Collings' (1950) survey of general practice in the UK. From 1952, data was collected on maternal mortality in England on a voluntary basis (Godber, 1976). This was important because this study focuses on reasons for inadequate care rather than simply recording incidences. This study formed the basis of similar studies in other parts of the UK and Australasia. It may also be seen to provide many of the characteristics of modern investigations:

• it focuses on improvement rather than recording current practice
• guidelines were produced to improve care
• compliance was voluntary
• standard data collection forms were used
• the study was evolutionary and ongoing.

Many audit initiatives have been driven by Government. In 1967, the Cogwheel report recognised that audit was 'a proper function for practising clinicians' (Williamson, 1973). In 1976 and 1979, Royal Commissions of Enquiry (the Alment (1973) and Merrison (1976) reports) reported the need for audit. However, the crucial step towards a national scheme came in 1984, when the UK Government signed the World Health Organization (WHO) health policy agreement which committed them to effective mechanisms for ensuring the quality of healthcare by 1990. A major reform of NHS management practices followed, culminating in the 1989 White Paper *Working for Patients* (DoH, 1989b) which made clinical audit a requirement for all doctors.

By comparison with other national healthcare systems, the UK has introduced audit as a quality procedure relatively recently. Audit activity within the USA may be considered to date from 1910, when a report by Flexner (cited in Roberts *et al.*, 1987) highlighted poor practice amongst USA surgeons.

However, until the 1970s, audit activity in North America, including Canada, was heavily focused upon cost reduction. In more recent times, there have been developments towards improving patient care. In the 1970s, California introduced occurrence screening (CMA/CHA, 1977). From this, clinical indicators were developed and used by the Joint Commission for the Accreditation of Healthcare Organisations (Shaw, 1988).

For the purpose of this analysis, it is worth noting that the UK did not generally adopt the occurrence screening approach. Early pilots (Bennett and Walshe, 1990) did not lead to widespread enthusiasm. The technique is based upon a view of quality assurance described by Garvin (1984) as the manufacturing view, or conformance to specification. This is popular in a culture where fear of litigation is a major factor. At the time in the UK, such fear was considerably less than in the USA. In the light of scandals, e.g. the Bristol scandal described below, such fear is now much more significant, and clinical governance will be formed partly by this cultural change. However, in 1990, the UK adopted a model closer to process improvement, based upon Denning's classical ideas (Denning, 1986).

Clinical audit 1990–1999

Clinical audit as a quality assurance mechanism

The original definition provided by the UK Department of Health (DoH, 1989c) was 'the systematic, critical analysis of the quality of medical care, including the procedures used for diagnosis and treatment, the use of resources and the resulting outcome and quality of life for the patient'.

The Department of Health definition set out the desirable characteristics of the audit process. Audit should be:

- systematic
- analytical
- concerned with the quality of care.

This statement also outlined the scope of audit activity. It should cover:

- procedures for diagnosis and treatment
- the use of resources
- the resulting outcomes
- the impact upon the quality of life of the patient.

The process of clinical audit was defined in the audit cycle (*see* Figure 10.1) which shows a remarkable similarity to the classical process improvement techniques (*see* Figure 10.2) pioneered by Denning (1986) and others (Juran, 1979).

Any quality mechanism should have two elements: quality assurance and quality improvement. Clinical audit as established within the UK NHS was designed to focus upon quality improvement. However, with many audits not completing the audit cycle, the improvement element was lost in many cases.

The practical reality of clinical audit

In a previous study (Gillies, 1996), the Oxford and Anglia region was used as a case study to investigate the implementation of clinical audit in practice. This study found the following.

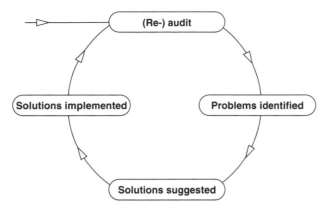

Figure 10.1 The clinical audit cycle.

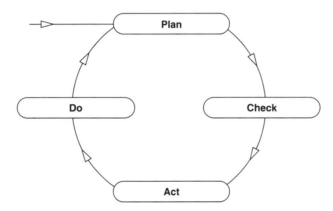

Figure 10.2 Classical process improvement cycle.
Source: Denning, 1986.

- The annual report (Anglia & Oxford RHA and NHSE, 1994) indicated that only 33% of all audits claim actual improvements and 46% claim to have produced guidelines or standards.
- Independent scrutiny of published audits, presumably exhibiting good practice, showed that 60% produced some improvement, but only 47% had either carried out a re-audit or indicated a commitment to do so.

In a more recent study, carried out in preparation for the introduction of clinical governance in the North Thames region (North Thames NHSE, 1998) 127 audit projects from 1997 were assessed.

- Of the 104 projects providing sufficient information for assessment, 50% had shown evidence of improvement and re-audit.
- A further 20% were incomplete and therefore could not lead to completed audit.

This indicates a similar level of effectiveness to the 1994 study. It should be borne in mind that this is the fraction of audit activity that is carried through to completion. It is a very small fraction of the clinical activity within the UK NHS.

The problems of clinical audit

There remains little evidence that clinical audit has had a widespread impact upon the quality of patient care. Clinical audit is not an effective quality assurance mechanism. It is not designed to be so. Its strengths lie in its local initiation and ownership.

The advantages of local control of audit projects should be seen in its role as a quality improvement mechanism, where local ownership should lead to greater acceptance of the findings and more readiness to change practice as a consequence. Further, local control allows audit to be carried out at different levels increasing the targeting of studies and the relevance of findings. Thus, the outcomes from clinical audit are specific isolated instances of improvements in patient care.

Clinical audit was introduced at the same time as other major management reforms into the NHS UK. The legislation establishing these reforms (DoH, 1989c) decreed that clinical audit became a universal activity and the principal mechanism of quality assurance within the UK NHS.

This has had positive and negative effects. Positively, it has made the collection of information easier with the widespread adoption of computers to meet the information needs of a broad range of activities from health screening to accounts. For example, amongst family doctors in the UK, the uptake of computers has risen from about 25% in 1985 to 97% in 1996. It has led to an appreciation of clinical audit as a quality assurance procedure rather than a research activity.

However, as a 'management' activity, it has been perceived with suspicion by many clinicians. In spite of local ownership and small-scale projects, some clinicians have viewed it as a nationally imposed programme and a threat to their independence. It is also perceived by some to have a hidden agenda of reducing costs rather than improving the quality of patient care. Sceptics such as these point to the experience of US doctors with the Professional Standards Review Organizations (Smitts, 1981) established in the 1970s. Much of this scepticism is attributable to the context of audit within the broader framework of management reforms introduced since 1987.

Clinical governance 1999–

Clinical governance as a quality assurance mechanism

Clinical governance is much more ambitious in scope than clinical audit. It emphasises quality assurance much more than quality improvement. It is intended to cover all aspects of the NHS. NHS documents describe clinical governance as a quality assurance process where quality assurance is defined as 'the use of a monitoring system to measure performance against quality standards' (North Thames NHSE, 1998).

Thus, the view of quality being proposed is conformance to a specification, and is much closer to the occurrence-screening model described above. Clinical governance will include assurance systems for:

- national screening programmes
- national vaccination programmes
- pathology services
- blood transfusion services
- radiation services
- patient pathway services
- patient charter monitoring
- patient records diagnostic coding
- health and safety procedures.

The impact of scandal upon clinical governance

Whilst clinical governance was being developed, the environment in which it was to operate was radically changed by a major scandal in paediatric cardiac surgery at Bristol Royal Infirmary. The longest enquiry ever held by the General Medical Council found that the deaths of 29 babies were due to the gross negligence of the doctors involved resulting in two doctors being struck off the medical register and a third being suspended.

The case generated a huge public outcry and undoubtedly shifted the UK healthcare quality assurance agenda. Smith (1998) argues that:

> 'The Bristol case', in which judgement was passed last week, will probably prove much more important to the future of healthcare in Britain than the reforms suggested in the White Papers. Reorganisations of the NHS come round with monotonous regularity, but changes on the wards and in surgeries are slow and often unrelated to the passing political rhetoric. In contrast, the Bristol case is a once in a lifetime drama that has held the attention of doctors and patients in a way that a White Paper can never hope to match.

There is evidence of other major catastrophes, e.g. major fires, shifting public policy by a major step change. Smith argues that this incident will impact upon professional practice in many ways:

- the need for clearly understood clinical standards
- how clinical competence and technical expertise are assessed and evaluated
- who carries the responsibility in team-based care

- the training of doctors in advanced procedures
- how to approach the so-called learning curve of doctors undertaking established procedures
- the reliability and validity of the data used to monitor doctors' personal performance
- the use of medical and clinical audit
- the appreciation of the importance of factors, other than purely clinical ones, that can affect clinical judgement, performance and outcome
- the responsibility of a consultant to take appropriate actions in responses to concerns about his or her performance
- the factors which seem to discourage openness and frankness about doctors' personal performance
- how doctors explain risks to patients
- the ways in which people concerned about patients' safety can make their concerns known
- the need for doctors to take prompt action at an early stage when a colleague is in difficulty, in order to offer the best chance of avoiding damage to patients and the colleague and of putting things right.

Smith's argument is that the lessons learned form this tragedy will be positive. However, if we focus on its impact upon the implementation of clinical governance then it has a number of specific consequences, which may be counterproductive.

1 It focuses upon a view of quality which is designed to prevent catastrophic failure rather than provide general improvement.
2 It has made it acceptable to scrutinise professional practice.
3 It emphasises a view that clinical governance is about weeding out 'bad doctors'.
4 It encourages defensive practice and therefore discourages innovation and improvement.
5 It may discourage doctors from operating on high-risk patients; all of the child patients in the Bristol case were in this category.

Current practice prior to the launch of clinical governance activities

Clinical governance represents a huge expansion in quality assurance activity for the NHS. It is unclear that the service is ready for this change. In a study into the readiness of 100 general practitioners (family doctors) (DoH, 1998b), a 52% response rate was achieved giving the following findings:

- 51% indicated that they currently used some form of risk management, e.g. complaint trend analysis, critical incident reporting, randomised prescribing checks, audits of minor surgery
- 45% currently contributed to their local audit activity
- 57% said that they had changed practice in the light of audit evidence
- 92% worked in multiprofessional teams
- 29% had attended training in clinical effectiveness
- 12% had carried out patient satisfaction surveys.

This study, from a self-selecting sample, i.e. the respondents, indicates that the level of activity is relatively static and that family doctors are not preparing in advance for clinical governance.

Another major area of concern in current practice in primary healthcare is availability of good quality information to carry out the monitoring process. The author has looked at the development of information processes to support a range of the New NHS reforms (DoH, 1997) including clinical governance. A five level maturity model, known as the General Practice Information Maturity Model (GPIMM), has been defined and described in Chapter 8. Within this model, five levels of information maturity are defined for practices with computers (Table 8.1).

The latest national data (NHSE, 1997) reveals that only 8% of practices achieve Level 5, while 3% are not computerised (Level 0) and 69% are at Level 1, leaving 23% at Levels 2, 3 and 4. Detailed work on coding and data quality with local practices (Ellis, 1998) shows that the majority of these practices are at the lower levels.

In order to implement clinical governance effectively, practices will need information processes and data quality defined as Level 4 within this model. Currently, it seems likely that a national audit would reveal that this applies to just over 10% of practices in the UK.

The problems with clinical governance

Clinical governance was introduced on 1 April 1999. There remain many barriers to an effective nationwide quality assurance scheme. The principal barriers to effective implementation seem to be:

- inadequate information and information processes
- lack of clarity of definition (Goodman, 1998)
- lack of training and preparation
- overemphasis on retrospective identification of catastrophic failure
- failure to build in quality improvement processes
- fear of a centrally imposed system.

Early indications based upon advice from regional NHS Executive offices to NHS personnel is that there will be an emphasis on checklists. A pilot regional project considered the care of diabetes. NHS staff were sent a three-page checklist of questions.

The checklist generates an ISO 9000 style quality management system that will ensure that the NHS has a documented procedure for almost everything. However, the experience in other disciplines (Gillies, 1997; Davis *et al.*, 1993) is that uninformed adoption of such systems produces bureaucratic and static systems which discourage change and hence improvement. Good practice in such systems is now considered to require more flexible systems that can be more responsive to the needs of the organisation. The ISO 9000 series of standards themselves (ISO, 1994) is currently under revision to facilitate such changes, and complimentary standards based upon process improvement are currently under development (ISO/IEC 15504) based upon the original Capability Maturity Model developed at the Carnegie-Mellon Software Engineering Institute (SEI CMM, 1995).

An evolutionary model for clinical governance

It is necessary to consider how clinical governance could be improved to make it more effective. Improvement in information processes can be achieved through the use of the author's GPIMM model (Gillies, 1998a, 1998b, 1999b). However, more fundamental changes are needed to achieve the following goals:

- reduce practitioner resistance
- increase the emphasis upon improvement rather than conformance
- integrate the currently disparate elements of evidence-based practice (EBP), research and development (R&D), and national guidelines.

In order to meet these goals, the author proposes a framework based on the evolutionary improvement and expansion of clinical audit. Evolutionary change will reduce fear, and basing activity upon existing good audit practice emphasises improvement and reduces antipathy to further change. This improvement can be achieved through the integration of EBP and R&D into the audit activity.

Rather than see clinical governance as a step change from clinical audit, the process of quality assurance and improvement may itself be seen as a process to be improved. This leads to a maturity model analogous to the original Capability Maturity Model and the GPIMM.

The maturity model for healthcare quality assurance within the UK NHS would be defined as shown in Table 10.1.

The use of an implementation strategy based on this approach leads to a process of evolutionary change and improvement rather than an attempt to impose a clinical governance system on an ill-prepared organisation.

Table 10.1 Healthcare Quality Assurance Maturity Model

Level	Description
1 Ad hoc	The audit process is carried out on an ad hoc basis; the activity is led by a few enthusiasts
2 Planned	Audit activity is planned to provide systematic coverage Basic monitoring is established to ensure coverage
3 Systematic	Processes for data collection, monitoring and improvement are defined and documented according to organisational quality assurance standards
4 Integrated	Full set of quality assurance procedures defined including data coding standards, validation and verification Quality procedures integrated with information and training strategies Use of IT to reduce administration burden and provide access to evidence
5 Automated	Automated data collection procedures and report generation mean routine effort is eliminated; effort focuses on improvement teams to ensure innovation

Conclusions

Quality assurance in the NHS is currently in a new phase. For the first time there is an attempt to introduce a systematic and comprehensive process of quality assurance. However, past experience in the UK and elsewhere, in healthcare and other disciplines, suggests that if political pressures arising from public outrage from scandals such as Bristol forces through an imposed solution without an evolutionary process of change, then the result will be a bureaucratic system with little impact on the quality of patient care.

The paper proposes an evolutionary model based on experience from other disciplines.

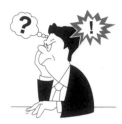

Questions to think about

Using the above paper as source material consider the following issues:

1 How does clinical governance differ from clinical audit?
2 How should the general public be involved in clinical governance?
3 What do you perceive as the key barriers to the implementation of clinical governance?

 Key points

By the end of this section, you should be able to:

1 Appreciate how quality assurance has evolved within the NHS.
2 Critique current measures adopted under clinical governance.
3 Use the GPIMM to analyse current clinical governance activity.
4 Advise your practice/PCO on their clinical governance activity.

11

The impact of scandal on clinical governance

Introduction

This chapter considers the impact of the Bristol scandal and subsequent inquiry on the introduction of clinical governance.

Clinical governance

To work through this chapter, you will need to read the following:

Goodman N (1998) Clinical governance. *BMJ*. **317**: 1725–7.
Smith R (1998) All changed, changed utterly. *BMJ*. **317**: 1917–18.
Department of Health (2001) *The Final Bristol Inquiry Report*. DoH, London.

As you are unlikely to read the complete Bristol inquiry report, try the 20-page summary!

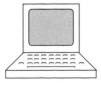

On-line resource
The Chapter 11 section of the website accompanying this book has links to both the Goodman and Smith articles and the Bristol inquiry website which offers the final report as well as a summary of all the supporting evidence.

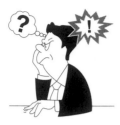

Questions to think about

1 Do you think that Bristol and other scandals will help or hinder the introduction of clinical governance?
2 Do you agree with Richard Smith's analysis?
3 Which parts of clinical governance will prevent another Bristol?

 Key points

By the end of this section, you should be able to:

1 Discuss the impact of the Bristol scandal on the introduction of clinical governance.
2 Discuss the impact of the Bristol scandal on the quality of patient care.

12

Decision making in healthcare

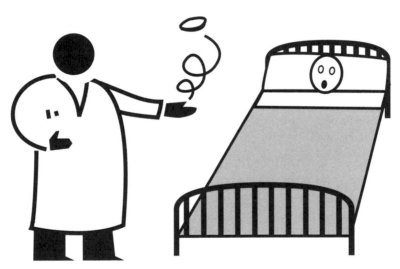

'Heads we stick a tube down your throat, tails we don't!'

Introduction

This chapter considers clinical decision making and the use of evidence-based practice. However, as physicians have been making decisions since the year dot and weighing evidence for almost as long, we shall attempt to set the subject in a reasonable historical context. The use of computers in attempting to support this process has been going on for longer than you might think.

A scenario

Consider the following:

A child patient walks into the consultation room with their mother. The doctor looks up and smiles at the patient. The patient and mother sit down. The doctor asks the mother what's wrong. She tells the doctor that the child has been feeling sick all night.

'Do you feel sick now?' The doctor asks the patient; she says 'yes'.

The doctor takes the child's temperature and looks down the child's throat. He checks the child's record on the computer. The computer tells him that the child is due for an immunisation.

The doctor reassures the patient and mother and sends the child home to bed to rest.

After the patient has left, during his coffee break, the doctor checks the PCT intranet to see whether there is any information about current infectious diseases.

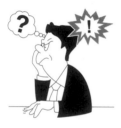 **Questions to think about**

1   How many actions in the scenario are intended to provide evidence for the doctor in making a decision?
2   What evidence is there in the scenario to assist the doctor in making a decision?

See my suggestions at the end of the chapter.

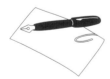 **Practical activities**

Rank the evidence in order of importance and relevance.

The doctor gathers evidence from many sources. He or she assimilates the evidence and weighs their relevance and validity in this case. This is what we pay clinicians to do. Any attempt at providing decision support must have the goal of improving this basic process. Please remember this throughout the rest of the book and use it as a benchmark for assessing all you will read.

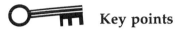 **Key points**

By the end of this section, you should be able to:

1 Analyse a consultation as a decision-making process.
2 Identify different types of evidence.

My suggested answers to the questions

Things that I consider to be actions to elicit evidence are shown in **bold**. Pieces of evidence themselves are shown in *italics*.

A child patient walks into the consultation room with their mother. The doctor **looks up** and smiles at the patient. The patient and mother sit down. The doctor **asks the mother what's wrong**. She tells the doctor that *the child has been feeling sick all night*.

'**Do you feel sick now**?' The doctor asks the patient; she says *'yes'*.

The doctor **takes the child's temperature** and **looks down the child's throat**. He **checks the child's record on the computer**. The computer tells him that *the child is due for an immunisation*.

The doctor reassures the patient and mother and sends the child home to bed to rest. After the patient has left, during his coffee break, the doctor **checks the PCT intranet** to see whether there is any *information about current infectious diseases*.

13

Development of evidence-based practice

Introduction

The movement towards evidence-based practice (EBP) in medicine is a global phenomenon.

The statement that all decisions should be based on evidence is glaringly obvious.

The case for EBP

First consider the case for EBP. The following is one of the best and most balanced expositions that I have found, from the University of Newcastle in New South Wales, Australia.

The practice of Medicine and Health Sciences requires decisions to be made about a range of issues.

Examples include:

- clinical decisions – about our patients, diagnostic and treatment pathways, best clinical practice methods

- research decisions – critically interpreting research, our research influences and directions, the questions we ask ourselves, applying research outcomes
- academic or continued professional education decisions – part of the life-long learning commitment, staying up to date, better care of our clients and patients
- health economic decisions – how can we better utilise resources, cost analysis, making limited resources go further.

Traditionally these decisions have often been made by individual healthcare professionals or by healthcare teams. In recent times patients have begun to take a more active role in the clinical decisions that affect them.

The end result of decision making is the effect that the decision ultimately has on clinical practice or work place standards, the diagnosis or treatment of our patients, or our research strategies, etc.

There are many influences that effect our ability to make decisions. Some of these influences include:

- our academic and clinical education as students and interns – Were we asked to manage problems and make decisions? Were we asked to evaluate our decisions? Were our decisions evaluated? Were we offered the opportunity to develop decision-making skills? Are we comfortable making decisions? What evidence did we collect and analyse in making our decisions? Are we able to ask questions of ourselves?
- our immediate clinical situation – local or situational policy and procedure, hierarchies of expertise and decision making, limited exposure to varied clinical situations. Are we allowed to make decisions that alter current practices?
- our own personality traits and limitations – in confidence, our flexibility as decision makers and our ability to reason in new situations
- the ethics of decision making – regardless of evidence what are the ethical judgements about the decision that needs to be made? Patients' rights and autonomy over decision making.

There are many aspects to decision making and many ways to make decisions. There is no one gold standard method of decision making, but there are best practice ways to gain the evidence that help support the decisions we ultimately make.

The concept of evidenced-based practice (sometimes known as evidenced-based medicine, or evidence-based healthcare) is that we should at all times attempt to clarify the evidence for the decisions we need to make, and apply an evidential approach to healthcare decision making.

It is a reasonably logical progression in modern medical decision making due to the improvements in research methods, the continuing development of informatics technology that can assist us in acquiring information, and the progression of the science of decision making.

Our personal experiences as practitioners in decision making

There was a time that all or perhaps most of us, medicine and health science practitioners, made decisions regarding the nature and extent of clinical procedures for our clients and patients by adopting the methods taught to us by our teachers and mentors.

Occasionally we might hear of a new method and attempt it once, reject it or accept it or modify it, and then move on either having changed our practice or by resuming old methods.

As we moved from one clinical appointment to another (consider this in your student role) we perhaps saw different approaches to doing similar things, and different and contrasting techniques and technology.

As technology developed and clinical practices changed we suddenly found ourselves having to evaluate new approaches.

> Which way was right? If there was a better way did this change in approach depend on the way I was going to apply it and who I applied it to?

During these times our evidence for what we did was based on our experiences and how we interpreted these experiences. Different people could have similar experiences but interpret them and apply them entirely differently. This led to ambiguous data being collected and expressed to those who would choose to listen.

We may also have faced, and perhaps still face, the dilemma of only experiencing some clinical situations infrequently. Patient presentations can be rare which means that we may not ever have the chance to gain a lot of exposure to these clinical situations. In these situations the collection of our experiences, or in this scenario our evidence, is limited.

> Were we right in what we did? Were we applying best practice methods?
> Were we keeping up to date?

Regardless of how, in retrospect, we would answer these questions, there is an element of personal experiences influencing the ways in which we make decisions. We all have our beliefs and biases. Consider the death with dignity debate or abortion issues or IVF issues.

There is nothing wrong with using our experience, our personal belief (anecdotal evidence) to help us in the decision-making process. There is nothing wrong with allowing our experiences to inform us.

But . . . we should be quite clear and understand that other health scientists are also having experiences with similar situations and that their data and their results may assist us.

If we combine all these experiences we begin to collect good evidence.

Experts and decision making

In most fields of endeavour, whether it be sport, the arts, or entertainment, there are certain people who become experts or are considered as experts in their particular field. The reason they become experts or are perceived to be experts is that they have shown a commitment to doing better, or they have acquired a higher level of understanding resulting in the better application of knowledge. Often experts conduct research or read current research methods and apply best practice protocols. They attend conferences and talk with their colleagues.

It could be considered that in Medicine and Health Science clinical practice there are clinical experts. Clinical experts tend to specialise in a field they find interesting. For instance in Medical Radiation Science (MRS) clinicians may become procedural experts in ultrasound or PET scanning or three-dimensional planning techniques, or they may become experts in designing and organising patient orientation and education programmes, or they may become experts in disease diagnosis and treatment. All fields of Medicine and Health Sciences have their experts.

Experts are a good source of information to help non-experts or generalists to make decisions. Because of their expertise they become a source of information. They help others gain better knowledge and understanding, and they can ultimately help assist other clinicians' patients.

Experts should be considered to be a source of evidence.

Patients and decision making

In issues concerning their welfare, patients deserve and should expect to be involved in the decision-making process. Patients have particular needs and desires concerning their health and information related to any procedures that they will be undergoing, and it can only be through discussions with the patients that this information can be established. Not all patients have the same goals in relation to their healthcare decision making. Some patients will defer all healthcare decision making to the practitioner, some will want to be partially involved, and some will want full control over the decisions to be made.

A clinician's role at times can be to explain all the diagnostic and treatment options available to their patients. They can be asked to act as advocates in helping make decisions for patients – because of their knowledge practitioners are well placed to suggest health strategies. At other times they need to work with patients to help make the best decision for each patient.

Patients are a source of evidence in relation to their healthcare needs and desires.

Research and decision making

Research is usually conducted in an effort to answer questions. The results of research mean that we have collected the evidence or data needed to help answer the question, or we have extended or increased our understanding of the issue.

Regardless of the research type, one thing that we must not do is to indiscriminately accept the results of research without carefully critiquing the source and methods used. The skills of critical appraisal are extremely important in allowing us to identify poor research from valid research, and therefore stopping us making the mistake of applying poor clinical methods.

No matter what research method is used, we should accept that decisions about patient welfare should at least have a strong grounding in research evidence. Where none exists we should attempt to collect it.

Health informatics and decision making

In the latter part of the twentieth century we have access not just to our close or immediate teachers, experts and peers, but also to the enormous wealth of information circulating in specialist and non-specialist journals, texts, CD-ROMs, at conferences, in tele-medicine, on the Web, etc. Technology and science developed health informatics and this conquered the tyranny of distance and isolation, the lack of experiences we may have with certain situations (others may report their experiences and research), as well as identifying paradigms for the collection of evidence.

The benefit that health informatics has on our clinical decision making and ultimately for our patients is that we can now access multiple sources of data, evaluate it, and if reasonable apply it to our own clinical situation. Using carefully applied critical reasoning criteria we can establish the most appropriate evidence we need for the variety of situations we face.

Our patients demand and deserve best practice methods. We should make the most efficient use of the funds that we have. We should use technology appropriately. We should add to the current evidence through carefully applied and evaluated procedures.

Therefore, due to technology the clinical decision making paradigm has shifted. We share experiences globally, and we benefit from shared experiences. We help create evidence. We use evidence as a dominant means of making clinical decisions.

Evidence-based practice and decision making

We have seen that modern EBP approaches embrace a variety of sources of evidence. Our experience, the experience of experts, and the views of patients all need to be considered when making decisions. The use of good valid research, carefully critiqued, supporting ours and our patients' decisions, means that we are implementing researched best practice approaches.

One definition for EBP is that it could be considered to be the application of appropriately evaluated sources of evidence to appropriately considered or matched clinical, research or academic situations.

It may mean replacing indecision, professional guestimates (gut feelings), or current practice, or what we have observed other practitioners doing, with considered and evidenced best practice.

Either way the use of EBP principles is one way of keeping up with the changes in the practice of our professions. It is not a panacea for clinical decision making but it can assist us greatly.

An alternative perspective comes from David Sackett, widely regarded as the father of modern evidence-based practice, writing in the *BMJ* (Sackett *et al.*, 1996; Straus and Sackett, 1998).

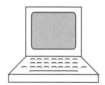

On-line resources
The Chapter 13 section of the website accompanying this book has links to these two *BMJ* articles.

The journal *Bandolier* has described the different types of evidence in terms of an evidential hierarchy.

The evidential hierarchy (*Bandolier*, July 1994, 6–5)

I   Strong evidence from at least one published systematic review of multiple well-designed randomised control trials

II   Strong evidence from at least one published, properly designed, randomised control trial of appropriate size and in an appropriate clinical setting

III Evidence from published well-designed trials without randomisation, single group pre–post, cohort, time series or matched case-controlled studies

IV   Evidence from well-designed non-experimental studies from more than one centre or research group

V   Opinions of respected authorities, based on clinical evidence, descriptive studies or reports of expert consensus committees.

This hierarchy is often cited in support of evidence-based practice, which strongly emphasises the supremacy of evidence-based over randomised control trials.

Some caveats

As often occurs, when a concept becomes dominant, some people will be quick to raise objections. To explore this theme, read the following studies:

McColl *et al.* (1998) General practitioners' perceptions of the route to evidence based medicine: a questionnaire survey.

Guyatt *et al.* (2000) Practitioners of evidence based care.

Lipman *et al.* (2000) Decision making, evidence, audit, and education: case study of antibiotic prescribing in general practice. Commentary: What can we learn from narratives of implementing evidence?

Young and Ward (1999) General practitioners' use of evidence databases.

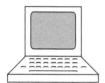

On-line resource
The Chapter 13 section of the website accompanying this book has links to these articles.

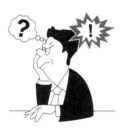

Questions to think about

1 What areas of healthcare are well served by an evidence base defined in terms of Levels I and II of the *Bandolier* hierarchy?
2 What areas of healthcare are not?
3 How much of your current practice is evidence-based? (This question can be applied to those in management as well as clinical positions!)
4 Can EBP be based on qualitative data?
5 How might we legitimise the use of less well defined evidence such as personal experience?

 Key points

By the end of this section, you should be able to:

1 Describe what evidence-based practice is.
2 Consider how much of your current practice is evidence-based.
3 Consider the pros and cons of EBP.

14

The context of evidence-based practice in the NHS

Introduction

There are two distinct approaches to decision making. The first is the approach of genuine decision *support*. In this approach, the clinician is in control, and aids are provided to assist them make the best possible decision. In the second approach, a degree of coercion is imposed to 'encourage' the clinician to make the 'correct' decision. The first is usually welcomed by clinicians. The second less so.

This 'encouragement' may be justified in a number of different ways.

- There is a vast amount of information out there these days. It is impossible for a generalist to know about it all. Therefore, it is necessary to make this available and encourage clinicians to access it.

There are big variations in care according to geographical area, and there is a need to provide equal quality of care across the UK, and that the care should be the best available.

This is the basis for much of the work going into quality initiatives in the NHS, such as clinical governance, decision support tools, e.g. PRODIGY, National Service Frameworks, National Institute for Clinical Excellence (NICE) guidelines, which are all based upon implementing the principles of evidence-based practice (EBP). However, opponents of these measures will point to the following counter arguments:

- There are large areas of healthcare where the evidence base is less than robust.
- Certain sectors of the population are under-represented in randomised control trials, e.g. children, old people and women who might be pregnant.
- If healthcare was able to be reduced to a set of algorithms, then we wouldn't need clinicians at all.
- Evidence from meta-analysis of randomised controlled trials (RCTs) will tend towards the lowest common denominator, and may hide variations due to genetic or environmental factors in a local population or individual.
- Whilst clinicians retain control, they can depart from guidance in appropriate circumstances. On the other hand it would be naive not to recognise that some clinicians are simply resistant to change and guidance.

EBP in the NHS

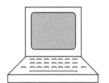

On-line resource
Read the following article:
The front line evidence based medicine project
accessible through the Chapter 14 section of the website accompanying this book.

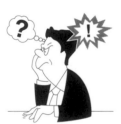

Questions to think about

This report was written in 1998.

1 Do you agree with its conclusions?
2 What has changed since this report was written?
3 What are the issues about applying this sort of approach in a primary or community healthcare setting?

 Key points

By the end of this section, you should be able to:

1 Discuss the pros and cons of decision support and the use of guidelines within the current NHS.
2 Identify barriers to the introduction of best clinical practice through EBP.
3 Identify the evidence in a particular area of healthcare.

15

Systematic review and meta-analysis

Introduction

In considering the quality of evidence upon which decision support and evidence-based practice (EBP) is based, the reality is that it is critically dependent upon our ability to combine evidence from a range of studies, through systematic review and meta-analysis. It is considered in this chapter specifically in the context of decision support and EBP.

Meta analysis

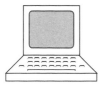

On-line resource
One of the key sources of information on evidence-based practice is the journal *Bandolier*, available electronically through the Chapter 15 section of the website accompanying this book.
    The following piece is taken from *Bandolier* and it may be found through the site.

Three recent papers on meta-analysis merit careful examination.

Predictive ability of meta-analysis

The first concerns the predictive ability of meta-analysis, namely the ability of a meta-analysis to predict the results of trials that may be done in the future.[1] The research workers calculated relative risks for 30 meta-analyses of different interventions in perinatal medicine and compared the results with the results of the largest trial done in each intervention. Twenty-four of the 30 meta-analyses correctly predicted the direction of effect in the largest trial.

A meta-analysis demonstrating protective effects of more than 40% from an intervention had a 60% probability of correctly predicting results of the same magnitude of the largest trial.

The authors confirm the finding that 'accumulative meta-analysis can help determine when additional studies are no longer needed and approve the predictability of previous small trials', referring to the classic paper of Lau *et al.*[2] But they emphasised that the results of meta-analysis are influenced by the readers of the technique, 'especially the way the trials are selected'.

This same theme was dealt with in two leading articles in the *BMJ* of the same week. 25 March 1995 was a big week for meta-analysis and the press.

An effective intervention that wasn't

The reasons for the leading articles in the *BMJ* was that in 1993 it was argued that magnesium treatment for myocardial infarction was, on the basis of a meta-analysis, 'effective, safe, simple and inexpensive'. However, the negative findings of ISIS 4, the Fourth International Study of Infarct Survival, contradicted the findings of meta-analysis.

ISIS 4 was a huge trial and offers the opportunity of comparing very large trials with meta-analysis. The authors of the leading article on misleading meta-analysis emphasised a number of points about meta-analysis:

* that more research is needed into the process of meta-analysis
* that registers of clinical trials are essential to reduce the risk of negative trials disappearing from view. The NHS R&D programme's project register system is designed to overcome this problem, at least for trials in the UK
* that results of meta-analysis exclusively based on small trials should be distrusted because 'several medium-sized trials of high quality seem necessary to render results trustworthy'

---

[1] Villar J, Carroli G and Belizan JM (1995) Predictive ability of meta-analyses of randomized controlled trials. *Lancet.* **345**: 772–6.
[2] Lau J *et al.* (1992) Cumulative meta-analysis of therapeutic risk for myocardial infarction. *NEJM.* **327**: 248–54.

- that the results of meta-analysis should be subjected to careful analysis to test the robustness of the findings.[3]

Too good to be true

The other leading article was written by one of the authors of the meta-analysis in question.[4] He and a colleague addressed the lessons to be learned from this changing conclusion, emphasising that there were two important lessons. The first was that a meta-analysis of small trials should not be a replacement for large, carefully conducted trials. The second was the need to be cautious of results that seemed too good to be true, and a more focused use of the lower confidence interval of risk reduction as a representation of what may be actually the clinical case – and is it useful?

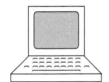

On-line resource
Now read the three papers from the *BMJ*,[3-5] available electronically through the Chapter 15 section of the website accompanying this book.

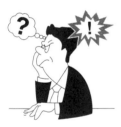

Questions to think about

1   What are the implications of these papers for the quality of evidence on which much decision support and clinical governance is based?
2   Read the more recent article on a similar topic, together with the ensuing debate in the electronic responses (Alejandro *et al.*, 2000). Consider the paper and the ensuing debate: does it change your opinion?

---

[3] Egger M and Smith GD (1995) Misleading meta-analysis: lessons from 'an effective safe, simple' intervention that wasn't. *BMJ*. **310**: 752–4.
[4] Yusuf S and Flather M (1995) Magnesium in acute myocardial infarction. *BMJ*. **310**: 751–2.
[5] Woods KL and Barnett DB (1995) Magnesium in acute myocardial infarction. *BMJ*. **310**: 1669–70.

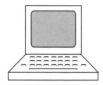

On-line resource
This paper from the *BMJ* is available electronically through the Chapter 15 section of the website accompanying this book.

 Key points

By the end of this section, you should be able to:

1 Explain the difference in evidence based on a large trial and a meta-analysis of a range of smaller trials.
2 Critique the quality of evidence presented to you based on systematic review and meta-analysis.
3 Explain why evidence may change over time.

16

National Service Frameworks

Introduction

One of the key issues within the New NHS White Paper has been the improvement of care in critical clinical areas, and especially the removal of inequalities due to geographical variations in care. The Government's answer to this problem is the introduction of National Service Frameworks (NSFs).

National Service Frameworks

The NHS document *A First Class Service* (DoH, 1998b) says the following about NSFs:

What do NSFs do?

NSFs set national standards and define service models for a specific service or care group, put in place programmes to support implementation and establish performance measures against which progress within an agreed timescale will be measured. Building on the frameworks for cancer and paediatric intensive care the first two NSFs are for mental health (published in September 1999) and coronary heart disease (published in March 2000). The first four NSFs are coronary heart disease, mental health, older people and diabetes. There will usually be only one new topic added per year.

Why are we developing them?

We need a systematic approach in order to establish service models that will ensure patients receive greater consistency in the availability and quality of services across health and social services. They will define explicit standards and principles for the pattern and level of services required.

Who is involved?

Each NSF is developed with the assistance of an expert reference group that will bring together health professionals, service users and carers, health service managers, partner agencies and others.

NSFs address the whole system of care and require partnerships with a wide range of organisations. These may include social care providers, the wider local authority, the voluntary sector, business and industry.

Now read the NSFs for mental health and coronary heart disease.

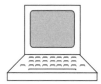

On-line resource
These NSFs are available on-line and may be accessed through the Chapter 16 section of the website accompanying this book.

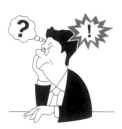

Questions to think about

1   What are the strengths of the NSFs?
2   What are the weaknesses of the NSFs?
3   Do you think that the NSFs represent 'cookbook medicine'?
4   How strong is the clinical evidence base for these documents?
5   What are the tensions or synergies with the organisational change within the system that have seen more locally-oriented organisations established, e.g. PCTs?

Information implications

More recent NSFs, including mental health, have had their own information strategies published with them.

Read the mental health information strategy.

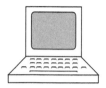

On-line resource
The mental health information strategy and *Information for Health* are available on-line and may be accessed through the Chapter 16 section of the website accompanying this book.

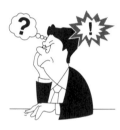

Questions to think about

1 What are the implications of this document for data collection in mental health?
2 What information tools might we be able to offer to help deliver the mental health NSF?
3 How does this strategy sit alongside *Information for Health*?

 Key points

By the end of this section, you should be able to:

1 Describe the nature and contribution of NSFs.
2 Define the role and usefulness of the information strategies produced to accompany them.
3 Discuss the implications for IM&T of these documents.

17

Technological support for evidence-based practice

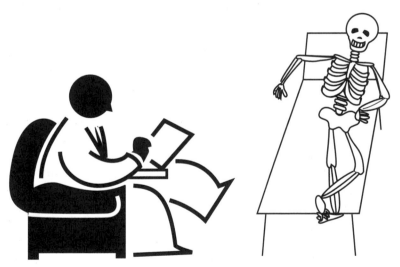

'My computer says that you're in a bad way, and that I need to measure your height, weight, blood pressure, iron count and perform a CT scan.'

Introduction

One of the major beliefs behind the push towards the use of clinical decision support is that the technology exists to enable best practice to be used consistently across the NHS. This is reflected in the following section from the *NHS Plan* document (DoH, 2000).

Support to redesign care around patients

Over the past few years the NHS has started to redesign the way health services work – in the outpatient clinic, the casualty department and the GP surgery. The work has been led by staff from across the health service and involves:

- looking at services from the way the patient receives them – asking their views on what is convenient, what works well and what could be improved
- planning the pathway or route that a patient takes from start to finish to see how it could be made easier and swifter – every step, from the moment a patient arrives at the practice, up to and including when they are discharged
- removing unnecessary stages of care – more tests and treatment are done on a one-stop and daycase basis
- identifying best, modern clinical practice – decisions are made about which professional should best carry out which functions. The result is a standard guideline or protocol for each condition.

Where this has been done the impact has been dramatic. It has resulted in improved services for patients. It has also resulted in improved productivity, made the task of caring for patients easier for staff, and in many cases it has released resources to spend on other services.

In North Tyneside General Hospital, the time the majority of patients spend in accident and emergency has been reduced from three to four hours to 36 minutes on average. This has been achieved by redesigning services for patients not needing to see a doctor when they come into casualty. Specially trained nurses assess patients in accident and emergency and make use of computer-aided decision support to provide the appropriate treatment. The use of nurses in this way enables doctors to concentrate on the patients who require medical treatment.

In West Middlesex University Hospital, services for patients with suspected prostate cancer have been transformed by redesigning the patient's journey. Under the traditional system, patients saw a doctor in an outpatient clinic, returned on more than one occasion for a number of tests, and then again for their results. The hospital team redesigned the process to allow clinical assessment and the tests to be carried out during a single visit, with the results available the following week. The time taken to identify a high risk for prostate cancer fell from six months to a maximum of 18 days.

Those places blazing the trail for this revolution in patient care demonstrate that the NHS can deliver modern, high quality, convenient services. Spreading best practice in the NHS however is often slow and ad hoc. Too many NHS organisations have been left to sink or swim, without external support to spread service redesign techniques.

In order to deliver this across the NHS, it is necessary to have:

- a strong evidence base that can be represented within a guideline or protocol
- technology in place to deliver the guideline
- staff trained in how to use the technology and deliver healthcare working in this way
- time to access the technology within the context of a consultation.

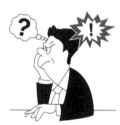

Questions to think about

1   Which of the above factors are the biggest barriers to you or your colleagues adopting this kind of technological support?
2   How can these barriers be overcome?

PRODIGY

Prodigy is the NHS's biggest decision support project for primary care. To help you evaluate it further, read the following accounts:

1   Read the evaluation report of the first (research) phase.

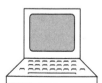

On-line resources
The evaluation report is available on-line and may be accessed through the Chapter 17 section of the website accompanying this book.

2   Read Iain Buchan's letter to the *BMJ* regarding the project:

BMJ (1996) **313**: 1083

Letters

Introduction of the computer assisted prescribing scheme PRODIGY was premature

Jacqui Wise writes about claims that have been made since an interim report was published on the computer assisted prescribing project PRODIGY. We are disappointed by the lack of statistical evidence in the report and thus by its lack of scientific integrity. PRODIGY, which was used by 137 practices, was evaluated over the period December 1995 to February 1996. In response to the question 'How much would you want to continue with PRODIGY?' 14 of the 86 respondents indicated that they would continue to use it, 32 indicated that they would continue if it was improved somewhat, 33 indicated that they would continue only if improvements were considerable, five selected the vague option 'some time in the future,' and two chose 'never again'. As opinions were solicited during the expected honeymoon period of the new system, these responses are downbeat.

Surprisingly, the results are reported as 'confirming desirability' of the system to general practitioners. The author of the report also claims that the system's 'effectiveness' is confirmed by the fact that prescribing costs (adjudged from the net ingredient cost per prescribing unit) for PRODIGY sites rose by 4.8%, compared with 5.9% for all other practices. This is reported as a 'relative reduction in the rise of expenditure of 1.1%'. Firstly, this is an absolute reduction and not a relative one. Secondly, there is no indication of the variance of this prescribing indicator for the groups compared; indeed, no statistical analysis is reported. The author lists a large number of evaluation methods, including a 10% poll of general practitioners by questionnaire, so considerable resources have been spent. If no reliable and statistically robust conclusions can be drawn then these resources have been wasted.

Perhaps it was misinformation that led the health minister, Gerald Malone, to make the specious claim that 'PRODIGY research has broken through frontiers in computer based support for general practice'.

Decision support in therapeutics is one of the most important areas for research into, and development of, clinical knowledge systems. In our opinion, the PRODIGY software was thrust prematurely into general practice systems as an active appendage to support decision making. This can alienate users by operating for some of the time as an 'uninvited guest' in the clinical decision making process. No computer can reliably predict what each user does not know; thus complementary active and passive systems to

---

support general practitioners' knowledge should be developed. In the case of PRODIGY, we believe that political initiatives have been misguided and that medicine has lost an opportunity to gather reliable evidence in computer assisted prescribing.

Iain E Buchan Research Fellow, Medical Informatics Unit
Rudolf Hanka Director, Medical Informatics Unit
David Pencheon Consultant public health physician,
Institute of Public Health, University of Cambridge
Peter Bundred Senior lecturer in primary care,
Department of Primary Care, University of Liverpool

Claims for PRODIGY continue to be impressive. Only recently, a New Zealand professor told me that 30% of UK GPs were using PRODIGY. PRODIGY has never been independently evaluated, and yet it is now part of every RFA-accredited practice system in the UK.

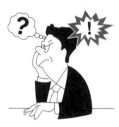

Questions to think about

1   Which of the factors mentioned above are the biggest barriers to you or your colleagues in primary care adopting PRODIGY?
2   How can these barriers be overcome?
3   See if you can find one of the 30% of UK GPs using the system and ask them!

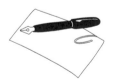

Practical activities

Visit the PRODIGY website. Look for the demonstrator and try it out.

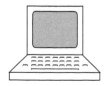

On-line resource
The PRODIGY website may be accessed through the Chapter 17 section of the website accompanying this book.

Key points

By the end of this section, you should be able to:

1 Describe the PRODIGY system.
2 Critique its strengths and weaknesses.
3 Evaluate the barriers to the wider adoption of this technology.

18

Evidence-based practice within clinical governance

Introduction

So far, we have considered the role of decision support as an aid to decision making. However, decison support tools may also be used to enforce certain actions on to clinicians. For example, consider the use of a computer to prescribe a drug. Three scenarios are possible within the context of a decision support role.

- *Free choice*   The computer may provide the clinician with the list of all possible medications relevant to the consultation.
- *Guided choice*   The computer may provide a suggested option, with alternatives. The basis for this guidance may be cost, clinical effectiveness in general, or based on knowledge of the patient, e.g. allergies or contra-indications with other medication already prescribed.
- *Mandated*   The computer may decide which medication the doctor may prescribe and not allow alternatives.

If this sounds like Big Brother, then it is, but we have already taken some steps in this direction. Consider the following:

1   One of the earliest areas of very simple decison support was the area of prescribing. Computerised prescribing guided clinicians towards the prescription of generic alternatives to expensive proprietary drugs.
2   PRODIGY now includes a component called PROFESS. This system is officially described thus:

PROFESS is an experimental project to determine the technical feasibility of collecting specific information from primary care practice systems, on a voluntary basis, for the purpose of providing a learning support system through an analysis service to subscribing practices. There is no compulsion to use the system, and the data is pseudonomised so that it is not possible to identify patients or clinicians. The primary purpose of the PROFESS system is to provide analysable information, for use by individual practices to reflect on their own practice information when compared, in an anonymised and secure way, with all participating practices. The analysis provision will help GPs to check, for example, data pertaining to their own patients in specific disease groups such as coronary heart disease (CHD) or diabetes. Another use for the system is as an adjunct to PRODIGY; although using PRODIGY does not automatically include the use of PROFESS. When used with PRODIGY, the system can provide information about the use of PRODIGY guidance, which could then be used to inform the future development of PRODIGY guidance in line with perceived patterns of use across all participating practices. The project is currently undergoing technical feasibility and is in the process of thorough evaluation. A government and professional ethics committee is also being set up to discuss and ensure the safeguarding of data use.

In spite of the careful language, this means that every RFA-accredited system has the capability to check up on the prescribing habits of the user. It remains to be seen whether the much vaunted safeguards are adequate.

Now read the paper – Clinical governance in primary care: knowledge and information for clinical governance (McColl and Roland, 2000).

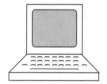

On-line resource
This paper is available on-line and may be accessed through the Chapter 18 section of the website accompanying this book.

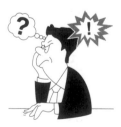

Questions to think about

Based upon this paper, and other documents read in previous chapters, where do you see decision support within clinical governance: free, guided, or mandated?

External factors

In reality, all but the most paranoid would agree that many initiatives in decision support are basically about guiding the clinician, rather than mandating. However, the use of the technology is taking place within a consultation which is currently within the context of the NHS. There are a number of a pressures on the clinician:

1 *Clinical governance*   The governance agenda is not necessarily fully appreciated by all the clinicians, but the push towards increased accountability can create an atmosphere of defensive practice.
2 *Litigation*   The current increase in no win, no fee litigation has certainly increased the volume and public awareness of litigation and this can also increase defensive practice.
3 *High profile scandals*   Public confidence in the medical profession has been eroded by a series of high profile scandals and a consequent increase in media scrutiny. This also creates a pressure towards defensive practice.

A defensive clinician is unlikely to over-rule a guideline, even when there are some indications that the individual patient may have specific characteristics that mean that the guideline is not the best possible care. In practice this means that a guided consultation may become a mandated consultation.

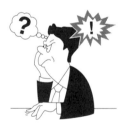   **Questions to think about**

1   In what situations should a clinician go against a guideline?
2   What action should they take to justify their actions in such a case?

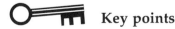   **Key points**

By the end of this section, you should be able to:

1   Categorise decision support as free, guided or mandated.
2   Identify external factors that impact upon clinicians' willingness to be guided by decision support tools.
3   Critique the role of decision support within the implementation of clinical governance.

19

NHS Direct: decision support in action

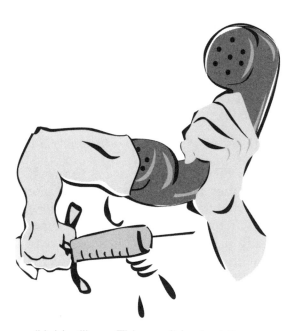

'Hold still . . . This won't hurt a bit . . .
still best if you go and see your GP in the morning!'

NHS Direct

One of the major planks of UK Government policy is NHS Direct. NHS Direct was first mooted in *Information for Health*.

> NHS Direct services offering telephone information and nursing advice will be available to the whole of England by 2000. NHS Direct will progressively develop a role as a wider gateway to the NHS including the piloting and development of appropriate telemedicine and telecare services in partnership with health and social care providers.
>
> Since 1992 the Health Information Service has run a telephone helpline for the public on a national freephone number. From the end of the year 2000 NHS Direct will be available in all parts of England providing quick 24-hour telephone access to health information and nursing advice. Work will be undertaken to look at the relationship between NHS Direct and the Health Information Service and to ensure that NHS Direct draws on the best practice of the Health Information Service. To help them in advising patients NHS Direct staff will be supported by a wide range of on-line databases and by a wide range of links to health services and other specialist helplines to ensure that, if the caller chooses, they can be seamlessly referred to other sources of advice and help.

This was expanded in *The NHS Plan: building the information core.*

> The focus of the current NHS Direct service is to provide patients with the information and advice they need to take better decisions about healthcare. This is an example of one of the principles of *Information for Health* in terms of using information and IT to enable patients to be better informed.
>
> The service is already up and running, has taken over three million calls, and is very popular with people who use it. In effect it has proved itself a different technical medium for delivering healthcare services.
>
> NHS Direct Online has been up and running since December 1999. It provides a wide range of accredited health information for the public and has received nearly a million visitors. It has established itself as one of the major UK health websites.
>
> NHS Direct is now going national. By virtue of the national nature of the NHS this will make it the largest service of this kind anywhere in the world.
>
> A central feature of NHS Direct has been the use of clinical decision support systems. Those systems have clearly underpinned the safety and consistency of advice given by nurses. NHS Direct has now completed a

national procurement of a national system which will be implemented across NHS Direct by April 2001. The system which will be controlled by the NHS will be known as the NHS Nurse Clinical Assessment System. It will also be available to use as a face-to-face decision support system in walk-in centres and A&E departments.

There are a number of planned developments. By April 2002 NHS Direct will use NHSnet to link its call centres together creating a virtual national call centre.

As highlighted in *The NHS Plan*, over the next three years NHS Direct will look to link up with other services providing the public with one-stop access to information, advice and where clinically appropriate a face-to-face consultation. Link-ups planned include out-of-hours medical services, dentistry, pharmacy and Category C ambulance calls. In linking up other services, NHS Direct will use NHSnet to share patient data, with consent, and contribute to the development of the patient-based electronic health record. As it starts to provide tailored services, including proactive outbound calls providing education and support for people with chronic conditions, NHS Direct will also need access to elements of those individual's electronic health records.

NHS Direct will be developing further its role in improving access to information for the public. This will include developments to NHS Direct Online including an e-mail inquiry service, development of further self-care material to support NSF priorities and, in partnership with nhs.uk, access to information about local services.

By 2004 NHS Direct will have launched a network of 500 public information kiosks providing wider access to the content of NHS Direct Online.

NHS Direct will be involved in the pilots of digital TV looking at the feasibility of delivering both the call centre services and content from NHS Direct Online through this medium.

NHS Direct exemplifies the need for a multi-channel communications strategy. As well as the call centre and on-line Internet services, there is a complementary written Healthcare Guide which supports patients by providing advice and guidance.

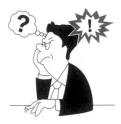

Questions to think about

1 Using the knowledge gained in this book and your own experience, think about three situations where NHS Direct might be helpful, and three where it might be harmful.
2 How reliable is the system at gathering accurate information from the patient or carer?
3 How easy is it for nurses to assess the accuracy of information presented to them over the telephone?

Now read the paper – How helpful is NHS Direct? Postal survey of callers (O'Cathain *et al.*, 2000).

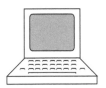

On-line resources
This paper, and the electronic replies to it, are available on-line and may be accessed through the Chapter 19 section of the website accompanying this book.

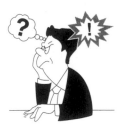

Questions to think about

1 How strong is the methodological basis of this article?
2 What does it tell us about NHS Direct?
3 Read the electronic replies to the article.

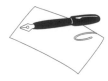

Practical activities

Visit the NHS Direct website and revisit your answers to the questions above based upon the on-line version.

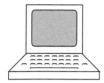

On-line resource
The NHS Direct website is available on-line and may be accessed through the Chapter 19 section of the website accompanying this book.

 Key points

By the end of this section, you should be able to:

1 Describe what NHS Direct is.
2 Assess it in terms of its use of clinical decision support systems.
3 Discuss its ability to deliver against the Government's stated aims.

References

Alejandro RJ, Moher M and Browman GP (2000) Systematic reviews and meta-analyses on treatment of asthma: critical evaluation. *BMJ.* **320**: 537–40.

Alment Royal Commissions of Enquiry (1973) HMSO, London.

Anglia & Oxford RHA and NHSE (1994) *Annual Report, 1993–94.*

Bennett J and Walshe K (1990) Occurrence screening as a method of audit. *BMJ.* **300**.

Boehm B (1981) *Software Engineering Economics.* Prentice-Hall, New York.

Bradley and Watkins (1989) Survey of equipment in general practice. *BMJ.* **299**.

Brown S (1988) Views of GPs in the Oxford region on microcomputing and collaboration with health authorities and family practitioners committees. *Journal of the Royal College of General Practitioners.* **38**: 115–16.

California Medical Association and California Hospital Association (1977) *Report on the Medical Insurance Feasibility Study.* Sutter Publications, San Francisco, CA.

Chisholm S and Gillies AC (1994) A snapshot of the computerisation of general practice and the implications for training. *Auditorium.* **3(1)**.

Collings JS (1950) General practice in England today: a reconnaissance. *Lancet.* 558–85.

Crombie IK, Davies HT, Abraham SC and du Florey C (1993) *The Audit Handbook: improving healthcare through clinical audit.* Wiley, Chichester.

Crosby PB (1986) *Quality is Free* (2e). McGraw-Hill, London.

Davis CJ, Gillies AC, Smith P and Thompson JB (1993) Current quality assurance practice amongst software developers in the UK. *Software Quality Journal.* **2**: 145–61.

Denning WE (1986) *Out of the Crisis.* MIT Press, Cambridge, MA.

Department of Health (1986) *Primary Care: an agenda for discussion.* HMSO, London.

Department of Health (1987) *Promoting Better Health.* HMSO, London.

Department of Health (1989a) *General Practice in the NHS: the 1990 Contract.* HMSO, London.

Department of Health (1989b) *Working for Patients.* HMSO, London.

Department of Health (1989c) *Medical Audit NHS Review Working Paper (6).* HMSO, London.

Department of Health (1992a) *Health of the Nation: a strategy for health in England.* HMSO, London.

Department of Health (1992b) *Getting Better with Information: an IM&T strategy for the NHS in England*. HMSO, London.

Department of Health (1997) *The New NHS White Paper*. HMSO, London.

Department of Health (1998a) *Information for Health: a national IM&T strategy for local implementation*. National Health Service Executive Information Management Group. HMSO, London.

Department of Health (1998b) *A First Class Service*. HMSO, London.

Department of Health (1998c) *Our Healthier Nation: the New NHS*. HMSO, London.

Department of Health (2000) *The NHS Plan*. HMSO, London.

Department of Health (2001) *The Final Bristol Inquiry Report*. HMSO, London.

Department of Health, Statistics and Management Information Division (1989) *Computing Survey, 1989*. HMSO, London.

Department of Health, Statistics and Management Information Division (1990) *Computing Survey, 1990*. HMSO, London.

Department of Health, Statistics and Management Information Division (1993) *Computing Survey, 1993*. HMSO, London.

Dyer C (1998) British doctors found guilty of serious professional misconduct. *BMJ*. **316**: 1924.

Ellis NT (1998) *The Sharing Information Project in Primary Healthcare (SIP) Final Report*. North West and South Lancashire Health Authorities, Lancashire.

Garvin D (1984) What does quality mean? *Sloan Management Review*. Boston, MA.

Gillies AC (1990) Survey of IT in the housing sector. *Proceedings of the ITLG Conference, Brighton*. HMSO, London.

Gillies AC (1991) *The Integration of Expert Systems into Mainstream Software*. Chapman & Hall, London.

Gillies AC (1992) Case studies. In: *Software Quality*. Chapman & Hall, London.

Gillies AC (1993) *A comparison of the computerisation of medical practice in the public health sector*. Interactive poster at HCI '93 conference, USA.

Gillies AC (1994) On the usability of software for medical audit. *Auditorium*. **3**.

Gillies AC (1995) The computerisation of general practice: an IT perspective. *Journal of Information Technology*. **10**: 75–85.

Gillies AC (1996) Improving patient care in the UK: clinical audit in the Oxford region. *International Journal for Quality Assurance in Health Care*. **8**: 141–52.

Gillies AC (1997) *Software Quality: theory and management*. ITCP, London.

Gillies AC (1998a) Computers and the NHS: an analysis of their contribution to the past, present and future delivery of the National Health Service. *Journal of Information Technology*. **13**.

Gillies AC (1998b) *Towards a maturity model for computer usage in general practice*. SIHCM '98, St Andrews.

Gillies AC (1998c) Can computers improve the health of the nation? *Journal of Health Informatics*. **4**: 147–53.

Gillies AC (1999a) *Information and IT for Primary Care*. Radcliffe Medical Press, Oxford.

Gillies AC (1999b) On the application of continuous improvement techniques to the problems of primary health care informatics. *Proceedings of the Third International and Sixth National Conference on Quality Management*. RMIT, Melbourne.

Gillies AC (2001) *Excel for Clinical Governance.* Radcliffe Medical Press, Oxford.

Gillies AC and Baugh PJ (1993) An evaluation of the computerisation of document production in a large public sector organisation. In: G Salvendy and M Smith (eds) *Human Computer Interaction: applications and case studies, advances in human factors/ ergonomics* (19A). Elsevier, Amsterdam.

Gillies AC, Ellis B and Lowe N (2002) *Building an Electronic Disease Register.* Radcliffe Medical Press, Oxford.

Gillies AC and Smith P (1994) *Managing Software Engineering.* Chapman & Hall, London.

Godber G (1976) The confidential enquiry into maternal deaths. In: G McLaughlin (ed.) *A Question of Quality.* Oxford University Press, Oxford.

Goodman (1998) Clinical governance. *BMJ.* **317**: 1725–7.

Guedon JC (1999) The digital library: an oxymoron? *Bull Medical Library Association.* **87**(1): 9–19.

Guyatt GH, Meade MO, Jaeschke RZ *et al.* (2000) Practitioners of evidence based care. *BMJ.* **320**: 954–5.

Hayes M (1985) Why don't more GPs use computers. *British Journal of Health Care Computing.* **1**: 19–23.

ISO (1994) *ISO 9000 Standard for Quality Management Systems.*

Juran JM (1979) *Quality Control Handbook* (3e). McGraw-Hill, Maidenhead.

Kitchenham B (1989) Software quality assurance. *Micropro Microcom.* **13**(6): 373–81.

Lipman T, Price D and Greenhalgh T (2000) Decision making, evidence, audit, and education: case study of antibiotic prescribing in general practice. Commentary: What can we learn from narratives of implementing evidence? *BMJ.* **320**: 1114–18.

Madely and Metcalf (1978) Doctors' attitudes to information systems: a survey of Derbyshire GPs. *Journal of the Royal College of General Practitioners.* **28**: 654–8.

McCall JA (1980) An assessment of current software metric research. *Proceedings of EASCON 80.* IEEE.

McCall JA *et al.* (1977) Concepts and definitions of software quality. *Factors in Software Quality.* NTIS, 1.

McColl A, Smith H, White P and Field J (1998) General practitioners' perceptions of the route to evidence based medicine: a questionnaire survey. *BMJ.* **316**: 361–5.

McColl A and Roland M (2000) Clinical governance in primary care: knowledge and information for clinical governance. *BMJ.* **321**: 871–4.

Merrison Royal Commissions of Enquiry (1976) HMSO, London.

North Thames NHSE (1998) *Clinical Governance, Discussion Paper (Revision 6).* Available from www.open.gov.uk/doh/.

O'Cathain A, Munro JF, Nicholl JP and Knowles E (2000) How helpful is NHS Direct? Postal survey of callers. *BMJ.* **320**: 1035.

OED (1990) *The Concise Oxford English Dictionary* (9e). Oxford University Press, Oxford.

Office of Health Economics (1989) *Compendium of Health Statistics* (7e). OHE, London.

Rigby M, Roberts R, Williams J *et al.* (1998) Integrated record keeping as an essential aspect of a primary care led health service. *BMJ.* **317**: 579–82.

Roberts JS, Coale JG and Redman RR (1987) A history of the Joint Commission of the Accreditation of Hospitals. *JAMA.* **258**: 936–40.

Sackett DL, Rosenberg WMC, Gray JAM and Richardson WS (1996). *BMJ.* **312**: 71–2.

Shaw CD (1988) Clinical outcome indicators. *Health Trends.* **21**: 37–40.

Shaw NT (2001) *Going Paperless*. Radcliffe Medical Press, Oxford.

Shum D (1992) The end of the beginning. *British Journal of Health Care Computing*. **10**: 24–5.

Smith R (1998) All changed, changed utterly. *BMJ*. **316**: 1917–18.

Smitts HL (1981) The PRSO in perspective. *NEJM*. **305**: 253–9.

Software Engineering Institute, Carnegie Mellon University (1995) Principal Contributors and Editors: MC Paulk, CV Weber, B Curtis and MB Chrissis. *The Capability Maturity Model: guidelines for improving the software process*. Addison-Wesley Publishing Company, Reading, MA.

Straus SE and Sackett DL (1998). *BMJ*. **317**: 339–42.

Watts R (1987) *Measuring Software Quality*. NCC Publications.

Williamson JD (1973) Quality control, medical audit and the general practitioner. *Journal of the Royal College of General Practitioners*. **23**: 697–706.

Young JM and Ward JE (1999) General practitioners' use of evidence databases. *MJA*. **170**: 56–8.

Index